DATES IN

OPHTHALMOLOGY

DATES IN
OPHTHALMOLOGY

DANIEL M. ALBERT MD, MS
University of Wisconsin, Madison, Wisconsin, USA

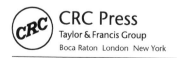

CRC Press
Taylor & Francis Group
Boca Raton London New York

CRC Press is an imprint of the
Taylor & Francis Group, an **informa** business

CRC Press
Taylor & Francis Group
6000 Broken Sound Parkway NW, Suite 300
Boca Raton, FL 33487-2742

First issued in paperback 2019

© 2002 by Taylor & Francis Group, LLC
CRC Press is an imprint of Taylor & Francis Group, an Informa business

No claim to original U.S. Government works

ISBN-13: 978-1-84214-113-7 (hbk)
ISBN-13: 978-0-367-39568-1 (pbk)

Visit the Taylor & Francis Web site at
http://www.taylorandfrancis.com

and the CRC Press Web site at
http://www.crcpress.com

Introduction

"Chronology provides the latitude and longitude of History. It is to History what the multiplication tables are to mathematics, what grammar is to literature, and what scales are to music. It imposes order on that which is otherwise anarchical." Such is Henry Steele Commager's description of the importance of *chronology* – the study of the arrangement of events in time. It is the purpose of this chronology, *Dates in Ophthalmology*, to present a concise listing of the chief personages, periods, publications, and events in the history of ophthalmology from ancient times onward through the centuries to the present.

There are, of course, many ways of looking at ophthalmic history: from the standpoint of the lives of major figures; of society and social impact; of subspecialties; of countries; of institutions; and of books. A chronology has the advantage of intersecting all of these, and demonstrating how ideas, discoveries, and technologies impacted on our specialty and how they crossed borders and oceans. It demonstrates the interplay of subspecialties, the changing pre-eminence of countries and cities; the explosions of creativity and generations of dormancy in various areas. In composing *Dates in Ophthalmology* I have been strongly reminded of how numerous and how diverse are the events and the men and the women who are responsible for shaping our specialty.

The focus of my review has been of Western medicine. While relevant events in Asia, the Middle East, Africa, and elsewhere are not intentionally omitted, I had limited material available to survey the historical events related to the development of ophthalmology in those parts of the world.

A chronology of dates, events, and periods in ancient medicine is largely conjectural and accuracy is often impossible. Starting in the 15th century, with the invention of movable type, a more accurate rendering of the activities of individuals, institutes and hospitals becomes feasible. The most reliable guide from this period up to 1900 is Julius Hirschberg with his encyclopedic history of ophthalmology, *Geschichte der Augenheilkunde* beautifully translated by Frederick C. Blodi. Julius Hirschberg's cardinal rule as an ophthalmic historian was not to write about the living and to say only good about the dead, ("De vivis nihil, de mortibus nihil nisi bene"), a rule he himself did not always follow. The first half of the 20th century has now come into clear perspective, and there is general agreement among ophthalmic historians as to significant contributions. Regarding the more recent history of ophthalmology, the myriad of facts with which one is confronted, dictates some degree of arbitrariness and assures omissions in attempting to identify what is important. Consequently, I believe that ophthalmologists and other browsers will find here most of the items that they expect as well as some surprises.

This work could not have been completed without the outstanding assistance of Kirsten Hope. She extracted, summarized, checked, rounded off, updated, verified, and completed these entries with intelligence, enthusiasm, and good humor. I was also most fortunate to have the advice and consultation of Richard Dortzbach in the arcane world of ophthalmic plastics and C.P. Wilkinson to lead me through the complexities of retinal surgery. Lenworth N. Johnson provided information on African American contributions to ophthalmology. The specific sources used in the development of this text are listed elsewhere. David G. T. Bloomer, the President and Managing Director of Parthenon Publishing, and Helen Lee, my Editor, were gracious, patient, and supportive. My wife, Eleanor Albert, remains my first and most exacting editor. Kevin Campbell assisted in editing the manuscript.

We often speak of *time* as a river. When we look at world history in recent times, the words of the philosopher Marcus Aurelius seem applicable: "Time is a river of passing events, aye a rushing torrent." However, for the history of ophthalmology, the American philosopher Henry David Thoreau, used a metaphor which I believe is more appropriate. "Time" he wrote, "is but the stream I go fishing in." I hope as ophthalmologists and other readers fish in the stream of *Dates in Ophthalmology* they will be rewarded with a greater understanding of the history of our specialty and of ourselves.

c. 3500 – 332 BC

As early as 3500 BC the Egyptians produced artificial eyes from metal and stone for use in mummies and statues. Their religion included DUAU as the god of ophthalmologists and MECHENTI-IRTI as the god of the blind.

c. 1950 BC

The Code of Hammurabi contains one of the earliest known records of ophthalmology. Sections relevant to ophthalmic practice are 196, 198, 199, 206, 208, 215, 216, 217, and 218. It contains the first mention of ophthalmic plastic surgery.

c. 1550 BC

The Ebers Papyrus was written. This is the oldest of several medical papyri, including the Hearst, Berlin, and Edwin Smith papyri (3000–2600 BC). These papyri consist mostly of compiled medical recipes, of which approximately 100 pertain to eye disease. The papyri included remedies for ectropion, entropion, and trichiasis.

c. 669 – 625 BC

The Assyrian-Babylonian practice of medicine was recorded on clay tablets. The medical system included the treatment of eye disorders.

c. 600 BC

PYTHAGORUS proposed the emanation hypothesis stating that vision was the result of a 'visual spirit' (pneuma) that came from the brain through optic nerves and into the lens. The retina's role in vision was relegated to guiding the 'visual spirit' and nourishing it.

500 BC

ANAXAGORA (500–428 BC), who founded the Athenian school of medicine, was born. Together with Alcmaeon, he countered traditional beliefs with his proposal that the brain was central to vision and other senses and to mental activity.

c. 500 BC

ALCMAEON OF CROTONA was most likely the first person to document the existence of the optic nerves, although he incorrectly described their structure. He developed a visual ray theory in which sight was achieved by an internal 'visual fire.'

c. 500 BC

HERODOTUS reported that women in Egypt performed skillful eye surgery using flint knives.

c. 500 BC

EMPEDOCLES suggested that 'visual rays' were responsible for sight. This theory was accepted by Greek students.

c. 460– 370 BC

DEMOCRITUS OF ABDERA was the first to describe the anatomy of the eye, noting two tunics of the eye, the 'fibrous tunic' comprising the cornea and sclera and the 'delicate tunic' composed of the uvea and pupil. He developed a rival theory of vision to that of Pythagoras, which held that each object constantly projects images of itself into the air.

c. 460– 377 BC

HIPPOCRATES founded modern medicine. He included details on the superficial anatomy of the eye and on the treatment of eye disease.

He also identified a third tunic of the eye: the retina.

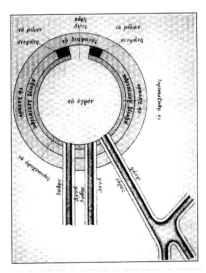

Structure of the eye after Hippocrates

431–404 BC	The disease trachoma was widely disseminated during the Peloponnesian Wars. The existence of trachoma was also noted in the works of Aristophanes, including mention in his play *Plutus*. Treatment for the disease included removing by abrasion the granulations that formed on the tarsal conjunctiva with Milesian wool wound around a thin stick of hard wood.
427–347 BC	PLATO combined the theories of Democritus and Pythagoras to reach his own vision theory. He believed that a pupillary 'inner light' and an 'outer light' emanating from a light source combined to make vision possible.
c. 371–288 BC	THEOPHRASTUS published *On the senses*, which discussed Alcmaeon's visual ray theory.
c. 340 BC	PRAXAGORAS wrote *About the flesh*. He described the optic nerve as a 'versal' extending from the coats of the brain through the bones into the eyes.
323–212 BC	HEROPHILUS OF CHALCEDON researched orbital anatomy, focusing on the optic nerve. He is believed to have authored a book on orbital anatomy, *Concerning the eyes*, which did not survive to modern times.
c. 290 BC	EUCLID, author of *Optika*, restated Pythagoras' emanation theory of vision. He believed that visual rays, in the form of discrete and divergent lines, emanated from the eye to an object and came back to the eye, resulting in sight.
c. 384–322 BC	ARISTOTLE developed a theory of vision in which an object emitted

rays toward the eye. The rays altered the medium, in ways specific to different object colors, which in turn altered the humors of the eye so that the color of the object could be viewed. He was the author of two books on the eye, which have been lost. He mentions the eye briefly in his *De parties animalium* and *Historia animalium*.

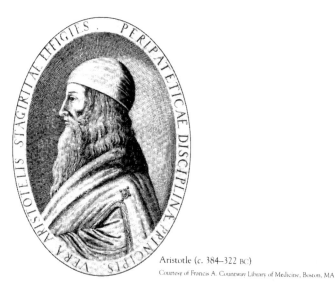

Aristotle (*c.* 384–322 BC)
Courtesy of Francis A. Countway Library of Medicine, Boston, MA

c. 250 BC	The Han dynasty in China produced an ophthalmology text entitled *Tzu-wu ching* (*The importance of needling*). This and later Chinese works detailed the use of acupuncture to treat many eye diseases.
c. 46 BC	The destruction of Corinth was followed by the migration of Greek medicine, including ophthalmology, to Rome.
25 BC–AD 50	AULUS CORNELIUS CELSUS wrote *De medicina*, widely considered the best surviving account of Roman medicine. It contains a considerable portion on eye diseases. Celsus also included the earliest directions for operating on cataracts. His discussion provides far more detail than previous descriptions of ocular surgery.
c. 100 AD	SCRIBONIUS LARGUS, a leading Roman oculist, compiled a 'formulary' of ocular diseases.
c. 60	Cilician physician, PEDANIUS DIOSCORIDES (AD 40–91) introduced the term trachoma in his *De materia medica*.
c. 77	PLINY THE ELDER (ca. 23–79) in his *Natural history* described water-filled globular glass vessels used as 'burning glasses' and stated physicians used them for cauterizing wounds. Pliny also stated that

Nero used an emerald as a lens to correct his nearsightedness.

c. 98–117   RUFUS OF EPHESUS lived during the reign of Trajan and was a skilled surgeon. Fragments of his writings contain descriptions of ophthalmic anatomy, including Tenon's capsule, the other membranes of the eye, and the optic chiasm. Rufus correctly described the position of the lens in the front of the eye, rather than the center, as was generally believed.

c. 200–500   SUSRUTA, the father of Hindu surgery, wrote a medical text describing techniques for rhinoplasty and one of the earliest accounts of couching and cataracts. This forms the basis of claims that couching was invented in India.

c. 200   PTOLEMY, author of the treatise *Optics*, supported the extramission theory of vision. He maintained that visual rays, in the form of an 'amorphous cone of radiation,' emanated from the eye to an object and returned to the eye and the object was seen by the viewer.

130–200   CLAUDIUS GALEN, a Greco-Roman physician who is considered the founder of experimental physiology, published *De usu partium corporis humani*, in which he reported six ocular muscles that control the horizontal, vertical, and rotational movements. He also wrote *Anatomy and physiology of the eye*, and *System of medicine*, in which he detailed cataract surgery. Galen swayed public opinion of ocular theory and ocular anatomy in his works, including *On the eyes and their accessory organs*. He was the first to promote superficial keratectomy (*abrasio corneae*) to attempt to restore transparency to an opaque cornea.

200   ANTYLLUS (a Greek physician) summarized the Greek concepts on the cataract operation and described a surgical procedure to correct ectropion.

304   ST. LUCY, the patron saint of the blind, was so named because she plucked out her eyes. According to one version, while being tried and tortured for being a Christian, she learned her prefect admired her eyes. St. Lucy removed her eyes and sent them to her torturer on a silver dish.

325–363   ORIBASIUS OF PERGAMON, oculist of Julianus Apostata, authored three works: a medical encyclopedia, *Collectanea medica*; a manual for physicians based on the encyclopedia; and a volume of household remedies for the layman.

525–605   ALEXANDER OF TRALLES was a widely traveled practitioner who eventually settled in Rome. His major work *Practica*, includes original material on ophthalmic diseases in Book II.

589–618   SHISH CHI during the Sui Sui dynasty wrote *Taos*, the first Chinese

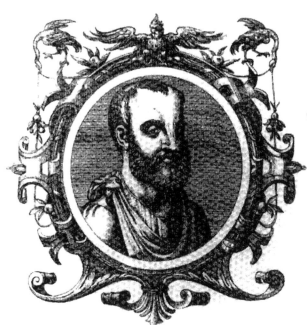

Galen (130–200)

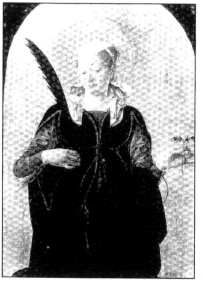

St. Lucy (300)

Schematic drawing of the eye after Galen

monograph on ophthalmic diseases, which included a description of 'double pupils.' The book was subsequently lost.

early c. 700   VAGHBATA I edited Susruta's work, which contained important sections on ophthalmology, dividing it into eight books. VAGHBATA II (eleventh century) further edited the work, compressing Susruta's work into one tome.

602–907   The *Yin hai ching wei* (*Essential subtleties on the silver sea*), written by SUN SZU MO from the T'ang dynasty, catalogued over 81 eye diseases. Some historians dispute both the date and author.

610   CHAO YUNG-FAN authored *Zhu bing yuan hou lun* (*On the origin and signs of all illnesses*). Comprised of 50 chapters, it contained several sections on eye problems and lists 51 eye afflictions. The eye was seen as reflecting the health of the internal organs, particularly the liver.

625–690   PAUL OF AEGINA, acknowledged as 'the last of the Greek eclectics and compilers,' wrote his *Epitome*. His sixth book provides the most comprehensive description now available of eye surgery in Greek and Roman times.

652   SUN SI-MIAO (581–682?) authored *Bei ji qian jin yao fang* (*Important prescriptions for urgent needs worth thousands in gold*). One-half the sixth chapter is devoted to ophthalmology and includes a description of presbyopia and an index of pathogenic causes of eye problems. In addition, Sun Si-miao lists oral and topical prescriptions for the treatment of eye problems.

732–1096   This epoch was classified 'the Era of Arabian Medicine' because Arab scholars preserved and augmented ancient Greek, Roman, and Alexandrian knowledge, which had become largely lost during the Middle Ages. This included optics and ophthalmology.

752   WANG TAO (ca. 670–755) compiled *Wai tai mi yao*, from a collection of 65 different works and was heavily influenced by Indian ophthalmology. He included 24 sections on ophthalmology and outlined the central importance of the eye in Chinese medicine.

c. 800–900   The 'Coptic Papyrus' was written, consisting of a collection of medical recipes, including many for eye diseases. This papyrus was discovered in 1892 written in Coptic, the language of the Christian Egyptians.

803–873   HUNAIN IBN ISHAQ, an Arab physician and medical translator also known as JOHANNITIUS, wrote and edited *Ten treatises on the eye* over a 30-year period, which gave his interpretation of the theories of Hippocrates and Galen. Hunain also authored the *Isagoge* and the *Questions on the eye*.

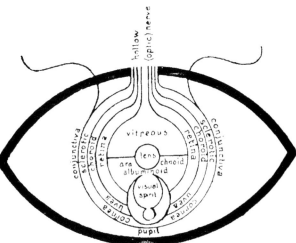

Eye after Hunain (803–873)

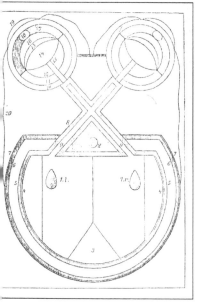

The optic chasm as depicted by Khalifah of Aleppo

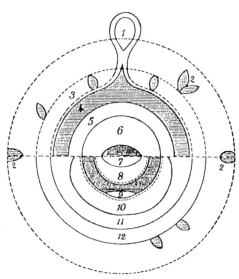

Eye after Rhazes

860–932	RHAZES was considered the most exceptional Arabian author and teacher. His medical encyclopedia *Al-hawi* (*Comprehensive* book) or *Liber continens* (*Content of medicine*) includes ophthalmic observations from his own practice.
d. 857	YUNA IBN MASAWAIH, a Christian physician at the court of Baghdad, produced the oldest known work in ophthalmology from the Arab world.
d. c. 870	ABI UISIF UA QIB IBN ISHAQ AL-KINDI was among the first in the Arab world to intensely investigate optics. He studied and translated the Greek literature on optics. Al-Kindi wrote *De aspectibus*, of which only a twelfth-century Latin translation, *On optics*, survives today. The theories of Euclid and Ptolemy shaped *De aspectibus*.
960–1279	Glasses were worn during the Sung dynasty, although their purpose is debated. They were probably introduced earlier.
965–1038	ALHAZEN OF BOSRA (ABU ALI AL-HUSAIN IBN HASAN IBN AL-HAYTHAM), known as the father of optics (both geometric and physiologic), was considered the most influential figure in optics in the medieval era. He supported the intromission theory of vision. Alhazen was the author of *Kitab al-ma nzir* (*Optics*), which comprised seven books focused on visual troubles. The most influential part consisted of a theory of the psychology of sight. He also wrote two smaller works that dealt with light and optics, *Perspectiva* and *De luce*.
984	YASUYORI TAMBA, a Japanese court physician, wrote a 30-volume medical text that was an aggregation of Chinese knowledge. The fifth volume included mention of 18 ocular diseases including cataract.
1025	ABU ALI AL-HUSAIN IBN ABDULLAH IBN SINA, or AVICENNA (980–1037), the Physician-in-Chief at the renowned Baghdad hospital, issued his monumental work, *Liber canonis medicinae* (*Canon of medicine*). His *Canon* was the Arabic text with the longest and most profound effect on ophthalmic practice. Avicenna also wrote *Kitab al-shia* (*Book of healing*), which had a segment on vision. Avicenna favored the intromission theory of vision.
c. 1100	In Salerno, Italy, where the medical education of women was permitted, a woman named TROTULA wrote a treatise on gynecology and midwifery. She is also credited with performing ocular surgery.
c. 1100	CONSTANTINE THE AFRICAN, a Benedictine monk at a monastery near Naples, produced *Liber de oculis*. Constantine coined the term *cataract*.
1100–1200	The early history of the Salerno school, the first lay medical school in Europe, remains obscure. Its curriculum included ocular sciences using Greek and Arabic texts but added little original information. One of the few examples of its medical faculty's supplementation was the *Regimen sanitatis salernitanum*. This text contained proposed cures

for eye diseases, including the use of blood, cautery, and rosewater.

c. 1000   *Tadhkirat al-kahhalin* (*Memorandum book*) was written by ALI IBN ISA (ca. AD 940–1010), known in Latin as JESU HALY. This became the classic textbook in Islamic and Christian worlds. The author was a Christian oculist and historian who practiced in Baghdad. Book I discusses eye anatomy and physiology, following along the lines of Galen's work. Book II deals with eye diseases generally and it includes some prescriptions. Book III discusses internal diseases of the eye and describes diseases.

c. 1000   ANMAR, a native of Mosul and a Moslem, wrote *Choice of eye diseases*. Considered the most original of Arabic ophthalmology texts of that period, it is a small book dealing with 48 diseases affecting the eyes. It included a section on cataract surgery and described a radical new operation involving the removal of cataracts by suction.

1025   The Montpellier school in southern France was established. By 1180 it was a university, and by 1137 it had a reputable medical faculty.

1088   ABU RUH, an Iranian, wrote *The light of the eyes*. The text was in Persian and described a total of 30 eye operations, including three methods of cataract surgery: couching with a needle; couching after opening the coats with a lancet; and suction.

c. 1200   DAVIDE ARMINO, a Salerno physician, published *Liber pro sanitate oculorum*. An apparent outgrowth of the *Regimen sanitatis salernitatum*, it was among the first to deal solely with ophthalmic diseases.

c. 1200   *The right guide in ophthalmology*, a discourse written by AL-GAFIQI (d. 1165) of Cordoba, covered ophthalmic practice and science, as well as providing substantial information on diseases of the brain.

c. 1200   MASTER ZACHARIAS, an oculist from Salerno, authored *Liber oculorum, qui vocatur sisilacera, id est secreta secretorum*. The book dealt with causes, diagnosis, and therapy for eye diseases and included a collection of prescriptions.

1111–1117   The *Shen ji zong lu* (*Comprehensive records of sagely help*) was assembled from all Chinese medical knowledge. Chapters 102–113 are devoted to ophthalmology and list hundreds of prescriptions.

c. 1250   BENEVENUTUS GRASSUS, from the Salerno school, was a very prominent ophthalmologist. A native of Jerusalem, Grassus went on to work and teach in Italy and France where he lectured at Montpellier among other schools. His text *Practica oculorum* discussed the anatomy of the eye, eye disorders, surgical practices, and treatments. Grassus was also the author of the widely studied book *De oculis*.

1175–1253   ROBERT GROSSTESTE of Oxford, and later Bishop of Lincoln, initiated a movement that developed a philosophy of optics strongly influenced by the traditional Platonic view. His theories were based entirely upon theology and were without the benefit of scientific examination or proof.

1186   LIU WAN-SU (1110–1200) of China authored *Su wen xuan ji yuan bing shi* (*Illness patterns originating in the mysterious workings* [*of etiology outlined*] *in the Su wen*). His section on eyes attributed all eye problems to excess heat, establishing his reductionist 'school of cooling.'

1189–1251   LI GAO, a Chinese theorist from the Son-Jin-Yuan era, authored *Lan shi mi cang* (*Secrets stored in the orchid room*). His ophthalmology section stresses the relationship between the eyes and the heart.

1240–1260   ALBERTUS MAGNUS (1193?–1280) was a natural philosopher who wrote extensively in the area of visual theory. He believed that vision was due to a change in the medium between the eye and the object, a change caused by the latter. He opposed the mathematically based theories of al-Kindi and Euclid.

1270   WITELO (VITELLO) (ca.1230–1275), born in Poland and educated in Paris and Padua, incorporated Alhazen's optics into a textbook that remained the standard textbook of optics from the thirteenth to the seventeenth century. This text formed the basis on which Johannes Kepler built his discussion of the retinal image using the analogy of the camera obscura.

1240–1260   ROGER BACON (1214–1294) formulated revised approaches to the study of optics. His visual theory rested on the background of Ptolemy and ibn al-Haytham and emphasized mathematics and the intromission theory. In his work Bacon devised laws of refraction and provided an explanation for rainbows. His texts include *De speculis comburentibue*, *De multiplicatione specierum*, *Perspectiva*, and his *Opus majus*, which drew on the works of Ptolemy, Euclid, and Alhazen. Bacon includes the first mention of lenses to correct vision.

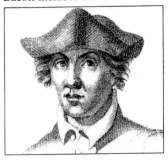

Roger Bacon (1214–1294)
Courtesy of Francis A. Countway Library,
Harvard Medical School, Boston, MA

c.1254–1324   MARCO POLO made mention of 'eyeglasses' in his account of his travels through China.

1213–1277 PETRUS HISPANUS (1213– ca.1277), prior to his selection as POPE JOHN XXI (1276), was a professor of medicine in Siena. Hispanus wrote *Liber de oculis* or *Breviarum magistri petri hyspani de egritudinibus oculorum et curis*, a compilation of some of the work of Constantine, Master Zacharias, and included an original tract on ophthalmology based on his own observations. It dealt with diseases of the eye, mentioned 'hardness of the eye,' and described operations for trichiasis, pterygium, and cystic tumors, as well as a collection of prescriptions.

c. 1260 KHALIFAH OF ALEPPO in Syria wrote *Khalifa ibn abi'l-mahasin*. The text was comprised of 560 pages and included figures regarding the eye and brain, a list of categories of cataract in table form, and a description of instruments and of a cataract operation. These manuscripts are among the first to include ocular illustrations.

1260 LOUIS IX founded in Paris the first institution for the blind called Hôpital des Quinze-Vingts, for crusaders who were blinded in Egypt.

c. 1270–1318 MUNDINUS OF LUZZI (ca. 1270–1318) taught medicine in the school at Bologna. Mundinus wrote *Anatomia*, which dealt with the anatomy of the head, and contained new details about the orbit. He described seven coats and three humors of the eye, perpetuating the errors of ancients. Mundinus also authored the book *Perspectiva*, which dealt with optics.

1250–1318 HEINRICH FRAUENLOB made early written mention of eyeglasses.

1282 JOHN PECKHAM (1230?–1292), Archbishop of Canterbury, wrote *Perspectiva communis* in which he described for the first time the action of concave refracting surfaces.

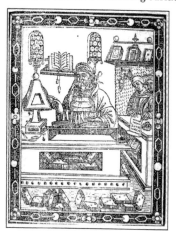

Frontispiece from *Perspectiva communis* (1282)
by John Peckham, the Archbishop of Canterbury

c. 1290	SILAH AL-DIN, a scientist and oculist from Hamat in Syria, wrote *The light of the eyes*, consisting of 178 leaves in folio, it covered optical theory and had an important chapter on cataract.
1295–1351	JEAN YPERMAN, called by some the 'father of Flemish ophthalmology,' authored *Chirurgie*, which included a chapter on ophthalmology.
c. 1300	AHMAD AL QAISI wrote *Result of thinking on the treatment of troubles of vision*. It was divided into 14 chapters according to the anatomical structures of the eye.
c. 1300	The Salerno school initiated special examinations for those who wanted to qualify in ophthalmology.
late 1300	Eyeglasses were invented in Italy. Though various people, such as SALVINO D'ARMATO DEGLI ARMATI, are attributed with inventing them, present-day medical historians persuasively argue that no single individual can be given credit for this invention on the basis of current available evidence.
c. 1342	DRAGIA, a woman of Slavic origin, was issued a medical license by the government of Venice in recognition of her skills in treating eye problems. She was one of six women issued Venetian medical licenses by *gratia* (i.e. without formal education).
1352	A portrait was painted by CARDINAL NICOLAUS of Rouen with a monocle set in a wooden frame. In the same year, TOMMASO DA MODENA painted a portrait of Cardinal Hugo of Provence with eyeglasses in wooden frames. Artists soon came to regard eyeglasses as a mark of respect, indicating the ability to read and denoting learning and influence.
c. 1400	NA FERRERIA, a woman who practiced in Prades d'Aillon in southern France became famous for her skills in treating eye disease.
c. 1400	KAMAL AL-DIN AL-FARISI (d. 1320) of Iran wrote *Tanqih al-manazir*, a commentary on ibn al-Haytham's *Optics*. This work became a landmark in the history of Islamic optics.
1363	The French surgeon GUY DE CHAULIAC (1298–1368) of Montpellier completed his *Chirurgie*, which cited Benevenutus, Galen, and Arab authors, as well as his own original observations. He included a detailed description of trachoma.
1443	The manuscript *De medicina* written by CELSUS was rediscovered in Milan after all copies were thought to be lost during the Middle Ages. It contained sections on the anatomy of the eye as well as ophthalmic pathology, therapeutics, and surgery.
c. 1448	GUTENBERG'S (c. 1397–1468) invention of the printing press

produced a mass-market demand for spectacles, as presbyopes and hypyopes required convex lenses to read the printed material.

1452–1519   LEONARDO DA VINCI played a large role in the beginning of modern anatomical studies, including those of the ocular structures. Da Vinci devised the earliest technique for embedding the eye for sectioning by placing it within an egg white and then heating the embedded specimen until it became hardened and could be cut transversely. He determined the retina to be the tissue essential to sight, correcting the previous belief that the crystalline lens played this role. Da Vinci wrote *Codex of the eye* (ca. 1508), which proposed the idea of contact lenses. This work is considered the precursor to modern contact lenses.

1475   The first printed drawing to depict spectacles is contained in *Rudimentum Novitorum, Lubeck: Lucas Brandis*. The illustration depicts an Alexandrian philosopher, Philo, wearing spectacles while seated at a desk.

1482   *Consilia saluberrima ad omnes egritudines noviter correcta et ad optimum ordine redacta* was published. Written by UGO DE SIENA (1376–1439), this was the earliest work to systematically organize medical cases and included descriptions of cataract, corneal diseases, and other eye diseases.

1491   GORDON DE BERNARD (or BERNARDUS), a University of Montpellier professor (1295–1307), published [*Lilium medicinae*] *In nomine dei misericordis incipit practia excellentissimi medicine dicta lilium medicine*. It was the first to advise the elderly to use eyeglasses as an aid for sight.

1493   HARTMANN SCHEDEL (1440–1514), the town physician in Nuremberg, published *Nuremberg chronicle*, in which he included one of the earliest printed illustrations of eyeglasses. A picture of glasses in *Ship of fools* by SEBASTIAN BRANT followed Schedel's work by one year.

1496   FRA TEOFILO ROMANO published *Libro de locchi morale et spirituale vulgare*. This is an Italian translation of a work written by PETRUS LACEPIERA and is the second book on the eye to be published.

1510–1590   AMBROISE PARÉ (1510–1590) made important advances in surgery, including his work in dermatochalasis. He advocated the use of Paul of Aegina's mask in the treatment of strabismus and used a speculum to lift the lid during surgery for pterygium and cataract.

1517   FRANCISCO LUCAS of Spain, followed by Italy's RAMPAZETTO and France's PIERRE MOREAU, designed devices for instructing the blind, including large wooden alphabet letters.

1521   AVERROËS (ABU AL-WALID MUHAMMAD IBN AHMED IBN RUSHD AL MALIKI) published *Paraphrasis De partibus et generatione animalium nuper ex hebraico in latinum translata per magistrum jacob mantinum*. It reviewed Aristotle's work of vision and opposed the Greek emanation theory of sight that was prevalent at the time.

1523   JACOPO BERENGARIO DA CARPI (1470–1530), a Bologna professor, gave the first accurate account of the conjunctiva.

1532   DAVID EDWARDES (1502–1542) of England, medical professor at Cambridge (1530), published *De indiciis et praecognitionibus*. This included an early mention of the optic nerves.

1534   The *Tetrabiblion*, an encyclopedic work by AETIUS OF AMIDA (502?–575?), was published in Greek by the Aldine Press in Venice. This printing included the ophthalmic section describing 61 eye afflictions. It is considered the best and most complete account of ophthalmology of its time.

1538   LEONHART FUCHS (1501–1566), botanist and physicist, professor of medicine at Tübingen, published *Tabula oculorum morbos comprehendes*. This was a 'fugitive sheet' or 'broadsheet,' which was designed as a substitute to costly textbooks for his students.

1543   ANDREAS VESALIUS of Brussels (1514–1564) moved far beyond Galen's anatomical teachings in his *De humani corporis fabrica*. Vesalius' ophthalmic anatomy studies made use of human dissection, and his discoveries included his revelation that the eye's anterior humor had the consistency of water. His depiction of the eye and orbit, however, was not entirely correct.

1546   JACQUES HOULLIER (d. 1562), at the University of Paris, published *Viaticum novum* containing three chapters on diseases of the eye.

1550   SIMONE PORZIO (1496–1554) of Naples wrote *De coloribus oculorum*. One of the earliest ophthalmology monographs, Porzio theorized on the reasons for different colored eyes and discussed Aristotle's and Galen's beliefs on the anatomy of the eye.

1550   GIROLAMO CARDANO (1501–1576) authored *De subtilatate rerum*, in which he suggested that touch could be used in place of sight for reading and writing. He introduced an early version of raised type.

1558   GIAMBATTISTA DELLA PORTA (1535–1615) of Naples published *Magiae naturalis*, which included a description of the camera obscura and his experiments in optics.

1561   GABRIELE FALLOPPIO (1537–1562) published *Observationes anatomicae*. This book rectified Vesalius' errors and added original anatomical observations, including accurate descriptions of the ocular muscles.

1561   PIERRE FRANCO (1506–1561), a barber-surgeon famous for his cataract and hernia surgery, authored four works that dealt in detail with eye diseases. He advocated the anterior approach in couching cataracts as

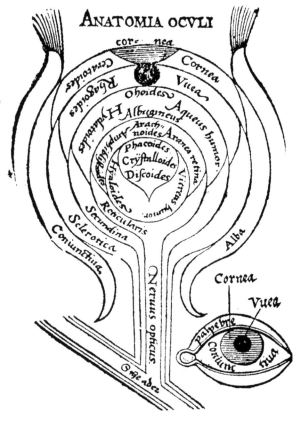

Schematic drawing of the eye by
Leonhart Fuchs (1538)

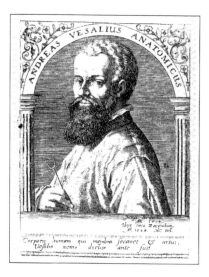

Andreas Vesalius (1514–1564)
Courtesy of Francis A. Countway
Library of Medicine, Boston, MA

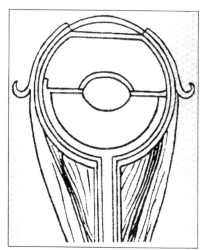

Schematic drawing of the
eye by Vesalius

it lessened the risk of injury to the eye. Franco's most influential treatise on cataract was published in 1561.

1564   PARACELSUS (1493–1541), professor at Basel, discredited the four humor theory and other theories of Galen. He categorized diseases on the basis of etiology and introduced mercury into the treatment of syphilis. His first collected edition on surgery, which includes material on the eye, *Opus chyrugicum*, was published in 1564.

1564   BARTOLOMEO EUSTACHIO (1524 –1574), anatomist at the Colleggia della Sapienza, in his *Opuscula anatomica*, advanced the study of anatomy of the visual system by describing the origin of the optic nerves. Eustachi produced a plate with an accurate rendering of the origin of the optic nerves. This was lost and not rediscovered until 1714.

1573   GIROLAMO MERCURIALI (1530–1606) of Padua wrote *De nervis opticis*, based on dissection techniques and observations transmitted to him through his correspondence with Costanzo Varolio (1543–1575) anatomist of Bologna. Variolo's work was the finest of its time in the area of optic nerve anatomy.

1583   GEORG BARTISCH (1535–1606), the 'Father of Modern Ophthalmology,' authored *Ophthalmodouleia: Das ist Augendienst*, the first 'modern' ophthalmic work, which detailed ophthalmic surgery and therapeutics, including the treatment of trachoma and enucleation for intraocular malignancy. Bartisch is recognized as the first to perform surgery to remove an entire cancerous eye from a living person. He also included sections on cataract couching and ptosis operations.

1583   PHILIP BARROUGH in England published *The method of phisicke*, an alphabetical compendium of all bodily complaints. He defined cataract as 'corrupt water, congealed like a corde, engendered of the humors of the eye.' Barrough distinguishes four types that can be cured by surgical procedures.

1583   FELIX PLATTER (1536–1614) of Basel wrote *De corporis humani structura et usu*. In this work, he concluded that the retina is the site where images of the extended world are formed.

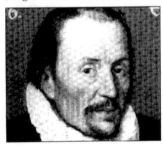

Felix Platter
(1536–1614)

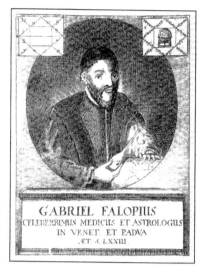

Gabriele Falloppio (1537–1562)
Courtesy of Francis A. Countway Library of
Medicine, Boston, MA

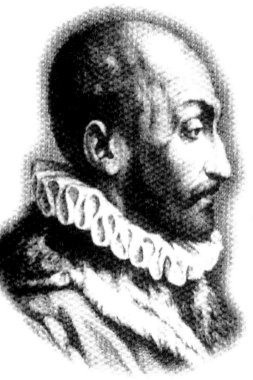

Giambattista della Porta
(c.1535–1615)

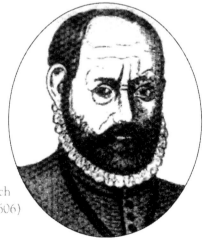

George Bartisch
(1535–1606)

1584	JACQUES GUILLEMEAU (1550–1613) wrote *Traité des maladies de l'oeil.* Guillemeau pioneered the correction of congenital eyelid coloboma.
1586	WALTER BAILEY (1529–1592/ 93?), Queen Elizabeth's physician and Oxford professor, published *A briefe treatise touching the preservation of the eyesight.* A popular treatise on the eye, this was the first vernacular work on ophthalmology printed in England.
1587	GUILIO CESARE ARANZI (1530–1589), professor at Bologna, demonstrated that the retina has a reversed image by means of his experiments with cow eyes.
1590	GIROLAMO MERCURIALI, now at Bologna, wrote *Praelectiones de morbis oculorum et aurium.* A large section was devoted to ophthalmology.
1590	GIAMBATTISTA DELLA PORTA of Naples described his invention of opera glasses.
1590	HANS AND ZACHARIAS JANNSEN of Middleburg, Holland constructed the first microscope.
1593	GIAMBATTISTA DELLA PORTA published *De refractione optices,* a treatise devoted to optics, which included valuable new observations on the eye as an optical instrument.
1596	EDWARD BREREWOOD (1556?–1613), an English mathematician and first Gresham College professor of astronomy, published the third section of his monograph, *Tractatus quidam logici de praedicabilibus et praedicamentis,* which discussed the eye. It is 63 pages in length and includes two full-page woodcuts of the eye.
1597	GASPARE TAGLIACOZZI (1545–1599) of Bologna published *De curtorum chirurgia per insitionem,* which revealed Sicilian secrets for facial plastic

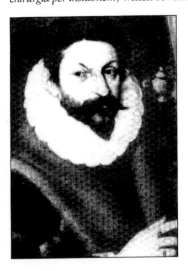

Gaspare Tagliacozzi
(1545–1599)

24

surgery, much of which is relevant to ophthalmology. He is best known for the rhinoplasty description, with autogenous grafting. Dieffenbach and Carl Ferdinand von Graefe later modified this procedure for use in blepharoplasty.

1598   ANDRÉ DU LAURENS (1558–1609), anatomist at Montpellier and physician to King Henri IV, published *Discours de la conservation de la veuë*. This is the second French monograph on ophthalmology.

1598   WILHELM FABRY (FABRICUS VON HILDEN) (1560–1624), a surgeon in Bern (1615–1634) called the 'Father of German Surgery,' published *Selectae observations chirurgicae quinque & viginti*. This was a compilation of 25 cases from his practice.

1598   MARIE COLINET of Bern (ca. 1598), wife of the great surgeon Fabricus von Hilden, became a celebrated surgeon in her own right. Fabricus credited his wife with being the first woman to suggest the use of a magnet to remove a metallic foreign body from an eye and stated that she excelled him as a surgeon.

1600   HIERONYMUS FABRICIUS AB AQUAPENDENTE (1533?–1619) published *De visione, voce, auditu*, which contained his treatise on the anatomy of the eye and orbit. His book *Tractatus de oculo visusque organo* (1601) presented a drawing of the eye in which the lens is placed directly behind the iris, close to the pupil. Unlike previous drawings, the lens was not separated from the pupillary margin by the 'cataract space.' This corrected the misconception of the location of the lens, which had been carried on since ancient times, and set the stage for an appreciation of the true nature of the cataract.

1602–1608   FELIX PLATTER of Basel made the first attempt at a systemic classification of diseases according to their symptoms. In *Praxeos medicae* he discussed the hardness of the eye in glaucoma and again emphasized that the retina was the true visual receptor of the eye.

1604   JOHANNES KEPLER (1571–1630), an astronomer and physicist born at Weil, Germany, published his influential book *Ad vitellionem paralipomena* (1604), which focused on ophthalmic topics. He opposed the popular belief that the lens is the essential visual organ and demonstrated that the retina is responsible for vision. Kepler also used his familiarity with ocular anatomy and optics to clarify how the eye functions.

1610   JOHANNES KEPLER, utilizing the optics of his telescope design, devised the basic light microscope, which utilized convex lenses and rendered a reversed image.

1651   THOMAS BARTHOLIN (1616–1680) of Copenhagen published *Anatomia*, a revision of his father's *Institutiones anatomicae*. A chapter with two plates is given to discussion of the eye. Bartholin was the first in modern times to mention sympathetic ophthalmia.

1611   JOHANNES KEPLER published his monumental *Dioptrice*, which included his important discoveries regarding the refracting telescope, refraction, and prisms. He included a more advanced theory of vision and described new findings regarding the anatomy of the eye. Kepler, who was myopic himself, developed an explanation for the cause of myopia. He gave the first report on spherical aberration, which he believed could be fixed with a 'hyperbolical form.'

1611   FRANCESCO MAUROLYCO (1494–1575) published *Di photismi de lumine*, devoted to optics. His work contributed to the development of aspheric lenses. Maurolyco's studies agreed with da Vinci's theories and those of Kepler that, contrary to Galen's teachings, the retina—and not the lens—was the seat of sight. Maurolyco also proposed theories on the cause of near- and farsightedness.

1611   MARCO ANTONIO DE DOMINIS (1856–1624) wrote *De radius visus et lucis in vitris perspectives et iride tractatus*. This provided one of the first modern explanations on the causes of rainbows. He also discussed the telescope and refraction by lenses.

c. 1612   GALILEO GALILEI (1564–1642) manufactured several compound microscopes utilizing both a convex and concave lens.

1613   FRANÇOIS D'AGUILON (1566/67?–1617) published *Opticorum libri sex, philosphis juxtà ac mathematicis utiles*. This exemplary treatise on optics summarized the works of Euclid, Alhazen, Witelo, Bacon, Risner, and Kepler. D'Aguilon reported on his own work on stereoscopic projections, describing these for the first time. D'Aguilon also made the first mention of the horopter and determined its role in binocular vision.

1615   SAMUEL FUCHS (1588–1630) published his treatise on physiognomy entitled *Metoposcopia & ophthalmoscopia*. Fuchs proposes a method for using the eyes and head shape as a means of assessing character.

1617   ORAZIO GRASSI (1582–1654), astronomer, physician, and professor of mathematics at Genoa and Rome published *De iride disputatio optica*, a brief work on rainbows and optics.

1619   CHRISTOPHER SCHEINER (1575–1650), a Jesuit mathematician, physicist, and astronomer, corroborated Kepler's conclusion that the retina was 'the seat of vision' based on his dissections of the eye. His *Oculus hoc est* included illustrations that were the most accurate to date regarding the eye and its relation to the central nervous system. Scheiner computed the refractive indices of the different eye components. He also described his pinhole test (Scheiner's test) for

Hieronymus Fabricius ab Aquapendente
(1533?–1619)

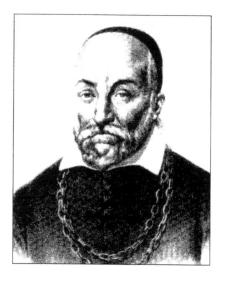

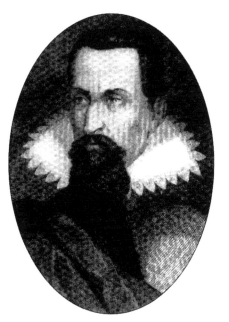

Johannes Kepler
(1571–1630)

Frontispiece from *Oculus hoc est* (1619)
by Christopher Scheiner

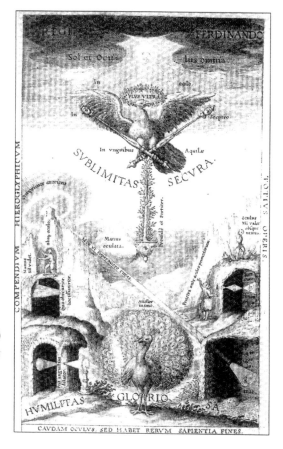

illustrating accommodation and refraction.

1621   WILLEBORD SNEL (1580–1626) described his law of optical refraction using cosecants.

1622   HENDRIK HONDIUS (1573–1648) published his classic Dutch work on optics and perspective, *Grondige onderrichtinge in de Optica, ofte perspective Konste*.

1622   CORNELIUS DREBBEL (1572?–1633) of Alkmaar, Holland, brought microscopes to England and subsequently constructed them there.

1622   RICHARD BANISTER (1570?–1626), an intinerant English oculist, published *A treatise of one hundred and thirteene diseases of the eye and eye liddes*, which consisted largely of a translation of Jacques Guillemeau's *Traité des maladies de l'oeil*. To this he added his *Breviary*, which contained the first modern mention of the hardness of the eye in glaucoma. The work also contained Walter Bailey's *A briefe treatise, concerning the preservation of eye sight*.

1623   BENITO DAÇA DE VALDÉS (1591?–1634), a Spanish inquisitor, issued *Uso de los antojos para todo genero de vistas*, regarded as the first book on spectacles. There are separate discussions according to genders. Women were given lenses that were twice as strong so that they could do precision needlework. He provides the earliest mention of cataract spectacles, stating the different strengths needed for distance and reading.

1626   FELIX PLATTER II (1605–1671) published an academic dissertation entitled *Theoria cataracta*, which popularized his uncle's previously ignored teaching that the retina was the true visual receptor of the eye.

1628   *En k'e ta chu'an (Most complete eyebook)* was written near the end of the Ming Dynasty. Consisting of six volumes, it covers 106 diseases, their treatment, as well as the couching and needling of cataracts.

1628   WILLIAM HARVEY (1578–1657) published *Exercitatio anatomica de motu cordis et sanguinis in animalibus (On the motion of the heart and blood in animals)*, his monumental study of the human circulatory system, which had relevance to most areas of medicine, including ophthalmology.

1629–1645   Russia's first known ophthalmologist, DAVID BRUHN, was employed by the regal court.

1632   BONAVENTURA CAVALIERI (1598–1647), a Jesuit professor of mathematics at Bologna, published *Lo specchio ustorio overo trattato delle settioni coniche*. This explained the optical principles of the sun's rays falling on mirrors and starting fires. He also demonstrated that a projection follows a parabolic trajectory. Cavalieri was the first to provide a formula for finding the focal distance for parallel rays of

Richard Bannister
(1570?–1626)

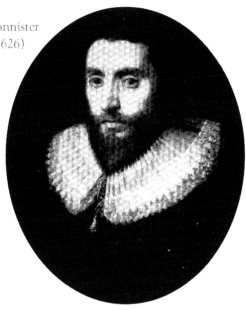

Benito Daça de Valdés
(1591?–1634)

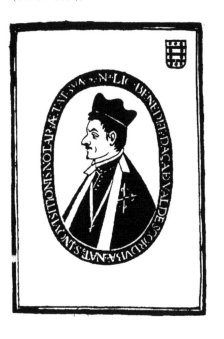

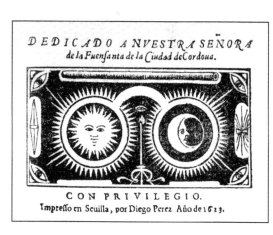

Illustration from *Uso de los antojos para todo genero de vistas* (1623) by Benito Daça de Valdés light for any convex or concave lens.

1632   VOPISCUS FORTUNATUS PLEMP (1601–1671), professor of medicine at the University of Louvain (1633), published *Ophthalmographia, sive tractatio de oculi fabricâ* in which he was the first to espouse the then-controversial optical theories of Kepler. Plemp also speculated that the clouding of the lens might be the cause of cataracts.

1637   RENÉ DESCARTES (1596–1650) published *Essais*, including his work on optics. He developed the Cartesian theory of the nature of light, rediscovered the law of light refraction, compared the eye to a camera obscura, and showed accommodation to be due to changes in the form of the lens induced by action of the ciliary processes.

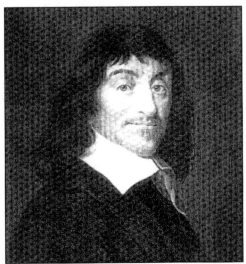

René Descartes
(1596–1650)

1640   PIERRE MOREAU, a notary in Paris, contrived several devices to enable the blind to read, including moveable leaden types.

1644   GIOVANNI BATTISTA ODIERNA (1597–1660), a professor of mathematics and astronomy at the University Ragusa, described the microscopic appearance of the eye of a fly in his *L'Occhio della mosca*. This was the first microscopic description of an eye from any species and represented an important milestone in the history of microscopy.

1644   WANG SHU PAO published *Yen k'e po wen (Hundred questions and answers of eye diseases)* during the Ch'ing Dynasty. It contains 111 questions and answers about many kinds of eye diseases.

1644   FU REN-YU published *Shen shi yao han (Precious book of investigation)* that discussed the concept of *kuo*, an anatomical feature of the eye that ensured enclosure and protection.

1645	JACQUES BOURGEOIS (1618–1701) of Paris described a new kind of spectacle lens 'being concave on the side nearer the eye and convex on the other in order to achieve effects intermediate between those kinds used hitherto.' This lens minimized 'aberrations, particularly marginal astigmatism.'
1646	POLYCARP GOTTLIEB SCHACHER (1674–1737) became professor of physiology and anatomy at the University of Leipzig. Schacher gave the first report of the ophthalmic ganglion and concluded that vitreous opacities were a possible source of *muscae volitantes*.
1646	ATHANASIUS KIRCHER, a Jesuit priest, published *Ars magna lucis et umbrae*. It included his studies on astronomy, light and lenses, and the camera obscura and the magic lantern
1646	A book on the condition of the blind was published anonymously in Italian and French and entitled *L'aveugle affligé et consolé*.
1648	EUSTACHIO DIVINI of Bologna (1610–1683) described his compound microscope based on Kepler's principles. An instrument of Divini's design was used by Marcello Malpighi in his observation of red blood cells.
1656	WEINER ROLFINK (1599–1672), a German surgeon, proposed that a cataract was an opaque lens and not a membrane between the lens and the iris, and he made actual anatomical demonstrations to verify this theory.
1657	MARIN CUREAU DE LA CHAMBRE (1594–1669), physician to Louis XIII and advisor to Louis XIV, published *La lumière*. He discusses the nature of light, refraction, and colors.
1657	THOMAS BARTHOLIN of Copenhagen published the second volume of his *Historiae anatomicae rariores*. It included the description of a diabetic woman who lost her sight before dying. He attributed her blindness to a cyst pressing on the optic chiasm, the first report of such an event.
1660	CARLO ANTONIO MANZINI (d. 1687) of Bologna published *L'occhile all'occhio dioptrica practia*. This was the earliest practical account of the contemporary methods of grinding and polishing glass for spectacle and telescope lenses. It contains an illustration of the first lens-grinding machine. Two chapters are devoted to the anatomy of the eye, vision, and its defects.
1662	ISAAC VOSSIUS (1618–1689) of Amsterdam, a classical scholar and polymath, published *De lucis natura et priprietate*. This is a treatise on the properties of light. Vossius attacks the Cartesian theories.
1662	NIELS STENSEN (1638–1686) of Copenhagen published *Observations*

anatomicae, quibus varia oris, oculorum, & narium vasa describuntur, novique salivae, lacrymarum & muci fontes deteguntur. Stensen, a physician and priest, made important contributions relevant to ophthalmology with regard to the anatomy of the glands, muscles, and the brain.

1662   RENÉ DESCARTES'S posthumous work, *De Homine*, was published, addressing the role of the nerve filaments and reflex action, as well as his ideas on vision. Descartes describes how light enters the eye and forms images on the retina, and then nerves carry messages to the ventricles in the brain. The pineal gland connects the mind and the body.

1663   JAMES GREGORY (1638–1675) of Scotland published *Optica promota*. In this work and in letters to Isaac Newton in 1672 he anticipated Newton in developing the design of the compound 'catadioptrical' telescope.

1663   JOHANN CHRISTOPHER KOLHANS (1604–1677) published *Tractatus opticus*, which included a discussion of the structure of the eye, principles of reflection and refraction, and the theories of light and color.

1664   ROBERT BOYLE (1627–1691), English chemist, physicist, and natural philosopher, reported on his work on 'color phenomena' in *Experiments and considerations teaching colours*. His studies laid the groundwork for Sir Isaac Newton's prismatic studies. He also discusses snow blindness and the iridescence of soap bubbles.

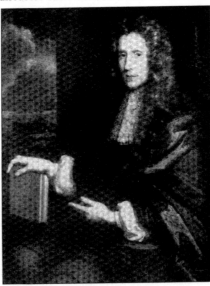

Robert Boyle
(1627–1691)

1664   ROBERT HOOKE (1635–1703), the London scientist, in the course of his studies on the resolving power of the eye, defined the measurement of the minimum visual angle.

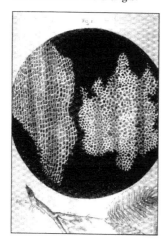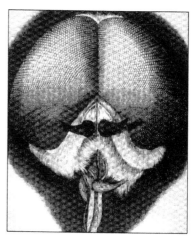

Illustrations from *Micrographia* (1665) by Robert Hooke

1664   THOMAS WILLIS (1621–1675), famed for his discoveries in neuroanatomy and neurophysiology, published *Cerebri anatome*. The description and classification of the cranial nerves superseded those of Falloppio and remained authoritative until replaced by Soemmerring's description. He also included the earliest discussion of the connection between visual field anomalies and pathologic alterations in the retina.

1664   DAWBENCY TURBERVILLE of Salisbury, oculist to Queen Anne and Samuel Pepys, gave the first report of color blindness to the Royal Society in London. He also reported extracting an iron splinter from the cornea with a magnet.

1665   ROBERT HOOKE of London published *Micrographica*. This was the first significant work on microscopy and describes the structure of cork as seen under a microscope. The book also displays his invention of a device to grind lenses and expounded an early version of the wave theory of light.

1666   HEINRICH MEIBOM (1638–1700), professor of medicine, history, and literature at Helmstädt, published *De vasis palpebrarum novis epistola*. This contains the first exact description of the sebaceous glands that bear his name.

1666   ROBERT BOYLE presented his further observational and experimental work on the nature of light and the perception of color in *The origine of formes and qualities.* In this work, he describes his 'corpuscular theory,' an early form of the atomic theory.

1667   HONORÉ FABRI (1606–1688), French physicist, mathematician, and Jesuit priest, published his work on optics, *Synopsis optica.* His observations on light and colors contributed to the science of optics.

1667   LUCAS SANTOMEE PETERS received authorization to practice medicine in New York. Peters, who was educated in the Netherlands, is regarded as the first African-American physician.

1668   *Heel-en Geneeskonstige Aanmerkingen* by JOB JANSZOON VAN MEEK'REN (1611–1666) of Amsterdam was published posthumously. Meek'ren invented a conical needle for the removal of hypopyon and performed an early enucleation ('extirpation') of the eyeball using the instrument devised by Bartisch.

1668   EDME MARIOTTE (1620–1684), a French physicist, gave the earliest description of the retinal blind spot. He was the first to recognize that there are only three primary colors, not the seven reported by Newton. He also appreciated that the red reflex was due to reflected light.

1668   ROBERT BOYLE in his *Disquisition about the final causes of natural things* presents observations on partially blind persons' abilities to perceive light and colors together with beliefs of the day regarding the causes of blindness and aids to vision. He also describes in detail a case of exophthalmic ophthalmoplegia.

1669   ANTONIO MOLINETTI (d. 1675), professor of anatomy, surgery, and theoretical medicine at Padua, published *Dissertationes anatomicae, et pathologicae de sensibus, & eorum organis.* It contains five illustrated chapters on disease and anatomy of the eye, and his plates illustrating the ocular muscles were a valuable teaching tool.

1670   FRANCESCO ESCHINARDIE (1623–1699), an Italian Jesuit mathematician and physicist, initiated the use of the Galilean type of telescope to aid patients with myopia.

1670   LANA TERZI, a Jesuit of Bresca, Italy, published an important book on the instruction of the blind.

1671   FRANÇOISE LASSERIE (1613–1697) was a French Capuchin scholar and instrument maker who wrote *La dioptrique oculaire* (1671) using the pseudonym CHÉRUBIN D'ORLÉANS. He discusses the effects of various kinds of glasses on the eye and explains his techniques for grinding lenses. He describes an early, stationary, compound microscope and provides the earliest description of the scioptric. This work is widely considered to be the best digest on seventeenth-century optical instruments and their construction.

1673 MARCELLO MALPIGHI (1628–1694) was physician to Pope Innocent XII and the anatomy professor at Bologna, Pisa, and Messina. He was a founder of histology and wrote *De ovo incubato observationes* and *De formatione pulli in ovo* both in 1673. These contained groundbreaking material on the embryology of the eye. Of particular importance was his meticulous description of the development of the optic vesicles.

1673 GEORG WOLFGANG WEDEL (1645–1721) of Germany was appointed professor of medicine at Jena. He published numerous medical works several of which deal with eye diseases, including *De nyctalopia* (1693), *De ophthalmia* (1713), and *De gutta serena* (1716).

1673–1723 ANTONIE VAN LEEUWENHOEK (1638–1723) was a shopkeeper and civil servant of Delft. Beginning in 1671, he constructed microscopes of increasing quality that allowed him to see the fine structure of the tissues of the eye in frogs and other animals. Van Leeuwenhoek gave early descriptions of the microsopic appearance of the optic nerve, the retinal rods, the lens fibers, and the lens and corneal epithelia.

1674 NICOLAS MALEBRANCHE (1638–1715) of Paris was a philosopher who devoted considerable attention to the study of optics. His principle work *De la recherché de la verite* (1674) contained a section on optics and vision.

1675 ZACHARIAS TRABER (1611–1679) of Vienna, professor of mathematics and Jesuit, published *Nervus opticus sive tractatus theoricus*. This encyclopedic and lavishly illustrated work is a classic on both physical and physiological optics. The book deals extensively with the anatomy and physiology of the eye and the properties of light.

1676 WILLIAM BRIGGS (1650–1704) of England authored *Opthalmo-graphia*,

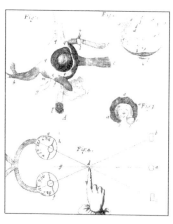

Illustration from *Ophthalmo-graphia* (1676) by William Briggs

an anatomy of the eye. Briggs provided the first description of the optic papilla and claims that this is where the sharpest vision occurred. He also presented his hypothesis of vibration to explain nerve action. Newton, a friend of Briggs, learned much about anatomy and physiology of the eye from the author.

1677
In *La vision parfaite* (1677), FRANÇOIS LASSERIE (CHÉRUBIN D'ORLÉANS) provided the first description of a binocular microscope and telescope he constructed to demonstrate his belief that a clearer image is created by using both eyes.

1678
FRANCESCO REDI (1626–1698), physician and counselor to the Medici, published *Lettera intorno all'invenzione degli occhiali*, in which he references a document on the invention of spectacles dated 1299. The authenticity of the document is doubted by modern historians.

1685–1686
JOHANN ZAHN (1641–1707) published *Oculus artificialis teledioptricus sive telescopium*, which promoted the use of telescopes to correct vision. He also invented 'the first refracting unit,' made up of a series of lenses, to be used for presbyopic and myopic testing. Zahn's 'refracting unit' is considered the precursor to the trial case. The last section deals with the grinding and polishing of lenses and construction of microscopes, telescopes, the camera obscura, and other optical instruments.

1685
JOHANNES MUYS (b. 1654), a surgeon in Steenwijk, Holland, published *Praxis medico-chirurgica rationalis*, which contained the earliest accurate illustration of the optic chiasm.

1685
PHILLIPPE DE LA HIRE (1648–1718), mathematician, physicist, and astronomer, in Paris, described a precursor to the modern contact lens designed to correct myopia resulting from curvature of the cornea.

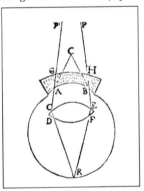

Philippe de La Hire's contact lens

1690
GOVARD BIDLOO (1649–1713) at the University of Leiden was the first to replace an injured eye with a glass prosthesis.

Johann Zahn
(1641–1707)

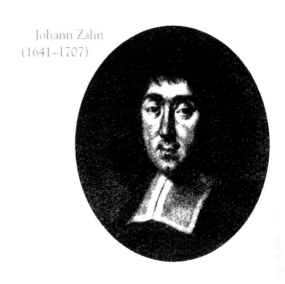

Frontispiece from *Oculus artificialis*
teledoptricus sive telescopium (1702)
by Johann Zahn, in Norton Library

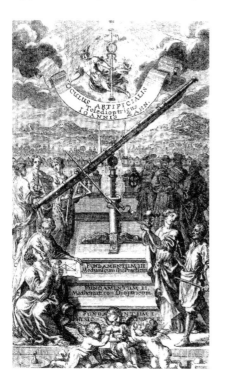

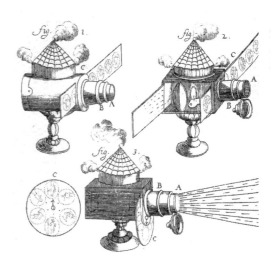

Illustration from *Oculus artificialis*
teledoptricus sive telescopium (1685) by
Johann Zahn

1690   CHRISTIAAN HUYGENS (1629–1695), a physicist of Den Haag, Holland, published *Traite de la lumiere* in 1690, which outlined his wave or pulse theory of light as opposed to Newton's corpuscular theory. Huygens also offered explanations of reflection, refraction, and polarization. In his posthumous *Opuscula*, he presented an exhaustive study of optics, 'Dioptrica,' and the theory of telescopes and microscopes.

1692   WILLIAM MOLYNEUX (1656–1698) of Dublin published *Diptrica nova*, the earliest treatise on optics in the English language. It contains many diagrams of mathematical propositions concerning rays that fall on convex and concave lenses.

1693   HERMANN BOERHAAVE (1668–1738) of Leiden, the premiere European physician of his time, was the first to correctly allude to the role the cerebral cortex played in vision. Boerhaave was the first to accurately describe the muscular fibers in the ciliary body, and he discussed Maître-Jan and Brisseau's observations regarding the true nature of cataract. His lectures on the eye were published posthumously in 1746 as *Praelectiones publicae de morbis ocularum*.

1694   NICOLAS HARTSOEKER (1656–1725), a physicist and instrument maker living in Paris, published his *Essay de dioptrique*. This contained a comprehensive review of the principles of optics, with discussions about the nature and origin of rays of light, the causes of color, the anatomy of the eye, the facts of vision, and the polishing and grinding of lenses.

1694   SIR WILLIAM READ (d. 1715), a notorious quack and former tailor and cobbler, began practicing as an oculist on the London Strand about 1694. He became a celebrity after the publication of his book *Treatise of the eye* (1706), which was actually a reprint of Richard Banister's 1622 book, *A treatise of one hundred and thirteene diseases of the eyes and eye-liddes*. His practice attracted the attention of Queen Anne, who knighted him, and later George I, who appointed him royal oculist.

1694   PHILLIPPE DE LA HIRE of Paris included in his *Mémoires de mathematique et de physique* (1694) studies on physiologic optics and the mechanism of vision, with particular emphasis on the physics of impaired vision.

1695   BERNHARD ALBINUS (1653–1721), while professor at Frankfurt, proposed an ingenious cataract needle. It was an elaborate instrument that, although it resembled a needle, when introduced into the eye, became on the pressure of an outside spring, a delicate pair of forceps.

1695   STEVEN BLANKAART (1650–1702) theorized on cataract surgery and suggested using forceps to take out a cataract. He included a chapter on ophthalmology in his popular text *Anatomia reformata*.

1695   GEORG ALBERT HAMBURGER mathematically defined the optics of hypermetropia.

1697   ANTONIO MARIA VALSALVA (1666–1723), a celebrated Italian otologist, is credited with introducing into Italy an accurate explanation of the seat and nature of cataract. Previously, it was believed that a cataract was a 'humor' located between the pupil and the lens. Valsalva disseminated Quarré's theory of 1643 that the cataract was an opaque, hardened, crystalline lens.

1700   FREDERIK RUYSCH (1638–1731), the Dutch anatomist, described in *De Oculorum Tunicus* the 'tunic of Ruysch,' or the lamina choriocapillaris. Other ophthalmic anatomical structures that he described included the vortex veins, ciliary nerves, and the iris's muscle fibers.

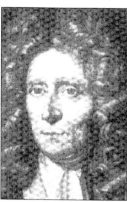

Frederik Ruysch (1638–1731)
Courtesy of Francis A. Countway Library of medicine, Boston, MA

1700   THEOPHILE BONNET (1620–1689) of Geneva's compilation of 3000 cases of gross pathologic anatomy, *Sepulchretum Anatomicum sive Anatomica Practica*, was published posthumously. The cases included 15 pages on eye pathology.

1702   JACOBUS HOVIUS (c.1678–1740) of Utrecht published his doctoral dissertation containing the first description of the circle of anastomoses (canal of Hovius) between the anterior branches of the venae vorticosae in the eyes of many mammals, but not usually in humans. It also contains the original description of intraocular circulation and the inflow and outflow of the aqueous, with primitive measurements.

1702   GEORG ERNST STAHL (1660–1734), a medical and chemical theorist while at the University of Halle, published his findings on the pathology, cause, and treatment of dacryocystitis. He also gave the first mention of lacrimal fistula and was the first to treat this condition on the basis of correct anatomical knowledge. Stahl explained that such fistulae have their origin in minor pathologic processes, which cause stenosis of the lacrimo-nasal canal. He treated this stenosis by threading a violin string through the upper punctum into the opening of the sac and then plugged the sac with healing balsams.

1704   JEAN MÉRY of Paris (1645–1722) provided the first description of the fundus in a living eye, while observing pupillary dilation in a drowning cat.

1704   SIR ISAAC NEWTON (1642–1727) published his great *Opticks*, describing his experiments with light spectra. He observed that lights of different colors have different degrees of refraction, and he provided a detailed discussion of light as a mixture of colors. This work contains the classical foundation and first full presentation of Newton's corpuscular or emission theory of light. Newton and Huygens are the two great founders of the modern science of optics.

1705   MICHEL BRISSEAU (1631–1717), the 'father of French ophthalmology,' published his studies that located cataracts as occurring in the lens.

1706   LOUIS DE PUGET (1629–1709) of Lyons published *Observations sur la structure des yeux de divers insectes et sur la trompe des papillons*. Puget described his microscopical observations of the eyes of flies, butterflies, grasshoppers, and crayfish, among others.

1707   ANTOINE MAÎTRE-JAN (1650–1725) of Méry-Seine, France reported that sight was possible without the lens. He confirmed Brisseau's discovery two years earlier that cataracts were hardened and opaque lenses, and he wrote of this in his *Traité des maladies des yeux*. Maître-Jan illustrated the lens structure as 'onion-like' and the vitreous as having a 'fibrous-fluid nature.' He also described in his book the use of chemical fixatives for pathologic examination of the eye.

1709   GEORGE BERKELEY (1685–1753), a philosopher and Bishop of Cloyne, published *An essay towards a new theory of vision*. In it Berkeley asserts the impossibility of the existence of matter independent of perception.

1709   PHILLIPPE DE LA HIRE of Paris explained why Jean Méry could see the details of the fundus oculi of a cat held underwater. La Hire concluded that the water obviated the refraction of light by the cornea, so that all rays leaving a given point from the fundus emerge from the eye not as parallel rays, but as divergent rays.

c. 1710   EDWARD SCARLETT (1677–1743), optician to King George II, devised

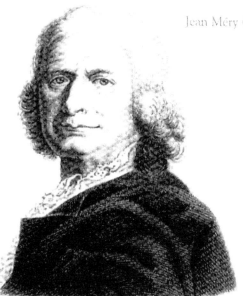

Jean Méry (1645–1722)

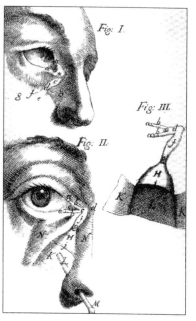

Anel's method of lacrimal
duct catheterization

Sir Isaac Newton
(1642–1727)

a system for differentiating eyeglasses based on their focal length.

1711   JOHN THOMAS WOOLHOUSE (1650?–1734), oculist to King James II, wrote of the possibility of iridectomy for the formation of an artificial pupil.

1711   J. BERNOUILLI succeeded in teaching a blind girl from Geneva to write.

1713   PETER KENNEDY (b. 1685), a London surgeon and ophthalmologist, published his *Ophthalmographia* that supported Brisseau and Maître-Jan's cataract theory and discussed diseases of the eye.

1713   DOMINIQUE ANEL (1679–1730), a French surgeon, described in his *Nouvelle methode de guérir les fistules lacrimàles* procedures by which the lacrimal duct was dilated and catheterized. He developed and used delicate probes (Anel's sound, Anel's probe) and syringes (Anel's lacrimal syringe).

1713   In his *The anatomy of the human body*, WILLIAM CHESELDEN (1688–1752), surgeon at St. Thomas' Hospital, described his procedure for iridotomy.

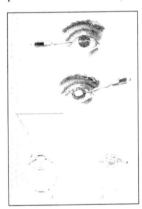

Illustration from *The anatomy of the human body* (1713) by William Cheselden

1714   DOMINIQUE ANEL published *Suite de la nouvelle méthode de guérir les fistules lacrimales*, which further outlined his procedures for lacrimal fistula surgery, with letters of support for his method from influential practitioners of the day, including Woolhouse, Méry, Fontenelle, and Lancis.

1715   BROOK TAYLOR (1685–1731), an English mathematician, published *Linear perspective* that, along with *New principles of linear perspective* (1719), presented the first complete enunciation of the principles of vanishing points.

1715   GOVARD BIDLOO, a distinguished anatomist at the University of Leiden, noted in a posthumous publication that internal phosphorescence was not the reason some eyes appeared to shine in the dark; rather it was reflected light. This view was not widely accepted.

1715   *Dr. Gregory's elements of catoptrics and dioptics*, written by DAVID GREGORY (1659–1708), was published posthumously. Gregory, professor of mathematics at Edinburgh University, corresponded with Isaac Newton and taught his new concepts concerning optics and mathematics.

1716   CHRISTIAN GOTTLIEB HERTEL (1683–1743) published *Vollständige Anweisung zum Glass-Schleiffen*. This reported on the idea of a 'split-lens,' the precursor to the bifocal. The same year, Hertel improved the microscope by adding a mirror, micrometer, and mechanical stage.

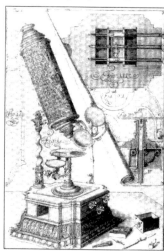

Illustration from *Vollständige Anweisung zum Glass-Schleiffen* (1716) by Christian Gottlieb Hertel

1718   LORENZ HEISTER (1683–1758), surgeon and anatomist at Helmstadt, published *Institutiones chirurgicae*, which contained an extensive section on surgery of the eye, the eyelids, and lacrimal system. Heister also supported the idea that cataract is an opacity of the crystalline lens.

1719   JOHN THOMAS WOOLHOUSE, now in Paris, in his *Dissertations sur la cataracte et glaucome*, attacked Brisseau, Maître-Jan, and Heister for their assertion that cataract is an opacity of the crystalline lens. He restated the old concept that it was a membrane between the iris and lens.

1721   JACQUES BENIGNE WINSLOW (1669–1760) introduced the term *iris* to describe the anterior portion of the uveal tract. He was also the first to point out that the center of the pupil lies not exactly opposite the center of the cornea, but slightly to the inner side.

1722   CHARLES DE SAINT-YVES (1667–1733) published *Nouveau traité des maladies des yeux* in which he described the removal of a cataract displaced into the anterior chamber. He also provides the first precise description of gonorrheal ophthalmia and the first descriptions of herpes zoster ophthalmicus and ophthalmic changes in variola.

1722   ANTOINE MAÎTRE-JAN of Méry-Seine, France, gave the first account of retinal detachment, observing it in the eyes of animals.

1722–1751   BURCHARD DAVID MAUCHART (1696–1751) was appointed professor of surgery and anatomy at the University of Tübingen in 1722. Mauchart published numerous valuable dissertations on a broad spectrum of topics in ophthalmology between 1722 and 1751.

1722   ANTONIO BENEVOLI (1685–1756), professor of surgery at Florence with a great reputation in ophthalmic surgery, published *Nuova proposizione intorno ala caruncola dell'uretra detta carnosità sopra la cateratta glaucomatosa*. Benevoli's work observes that the cause of cataract is loss of transparency of the lens rather than the formation of a membrane in the vitreous body. For this observation, Benevoli was accused of plagiarizing Heister.

1723   JEAN LOUIS PETIT (1674–1750) of Paris was the first to explain the conduction of tears from the conjunctival sac into the lacrimal passages and onto the nose. He invented a new operation for lacrimal fistulas, opening the passages with probes and then irrigating with lukewarm water through a syringe. He studied and theorized about the causes of cataract and developed an improved couching technique. Petit also carried out studies on the curvature of the lens.

1725   EDMUND CULPEPPER improved the microscope with his invention of the concave illuminating mirror.

1725   BENJAMIN MARTIN (1704–1782), a self-taught London mathematician and instrument maker, began his career as a teacher, traveling lecturer, and author, informing the public about Newtonian optics, the principles of microscopes and telescopes, and the use and construction of spectacles.

1726   JOHN WOOLHOUSE, living in Paris, declared on the basis of his experience that fragmentation should be performed when possible in the treatment of cataract rather than dislocation by the usual couching technique.

1726   JOHANN ZACHARIAS PLATNER (1694–1747), professor of surgery at Leipzig, described a method for extirpation of the lacrimal sac (dacryocystectomy) that he attributed to his teacher, John Woolhouse.

1728   HENRY PEMBERTON (1694–1771) of London published A *view of Sir*

Isaac Newton's philosophy. Pemberton was the first to use the terms *accommodate* and *accommodation* in reference to the action of the eye in changing from distant to near vision. He assumed that accommodation was produced by a change in the lens surface and believed that the lens fibers were muscular in nature.

1728   JACQUES DAVIEL (1696–1762), a French surgeon who was later the inventor of cataract extraction, limited his practice to the treatment of diseases of the eye.

1728   EDWARD SCARLETT, optician to George II, invented the modern method of keeping eyeglasses on the nose by affixing temples to the spectacles.

1729   FRANÇOIS POURFOUT DU PETIT (1664–1741), a surgeon in Paris, published *Lettre de M. Petit*, contradicting Phillippe Hecquet's monograph of 1727, which stated that the lens lay in the center of the eyeball and the cataract is a membrane. Petit correctly stated the anatomy and pathology of the lens and cataract. He provided accurate measurements of the human eye and described his method for cataract surgery, making an incision in the cornea and using a silver spoon to scoop out the cataract. Petit accurately depicted the posterior chamber and initiated frozen ocular sections.

1729   BENEDICT DUDDELL, an English ophthalmologist about whom little is known, described the posterior 'glass' membrane of the cornea in his book *A treatise of the diseases of the horny-coat of the eye, and the various kinds of cataract.*

1733   ROGER BACON'S seminal medieval scientific work, *Opus majus*, originally written in manuscript form in 1266–1267, was published. Part 5, the *Perspectiva*, deals with physiological optics and states the laws of reflection and refraction.

1735   ALEXANDER MONRO, *primus*, (1697–1767), the founder of a dynasty of anatomy teachers in Edinburgh, published an article on lacrimal diseases. He described the use of a probe in the diagnosis and treatment of lacrimal disease and in some cases removal of the lacrimal sac. This was one of the earliest works to suggest such treatment.

1738   JOHANN NATHANAEL LIEBERKUHN (1711–1756) designed a better reflector for microscopes that improved on the reflectors of Descartes and Leeuwenhoek.

1738   JOHN TAYLOR (1703–1772), often called CHEVALIER TAYLOR, a notorious quack-oculist, did, however, develop a partial understanding of the causes and potential surgical treatment of strabismus. This is mentioned in *Le mechanisme ou le nouveau traité de l'anatomie du globe de l'oeuil.*

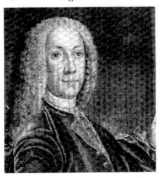

Portrait of John Taylor from
Le mechanisme ou le nouveau traité de l'anatomie du globe de l'oeuil (1738)

1738   ROBERT SMITH (1689–1768), a physicist and Plumian professor of astronomy at Trinity College, Cambridge, published *A compleat system of optics*. This work helped establish the particulate theory of light. Smith offers a comprehensive set of geometric propositions for the computation of focus, location, magnification, brightness, and aberrations of systems of lenses and mirrors and gives instructions for the construction of optical instruments.

1738   JAMES JURIN (1684–1750), a student of Newton and a London physician, published *An essay upon distinct and indistinct vision*, which discusses the phenomena of vision, the limits of perfect vision, and changes in the eyes. Jurins work was issued with Smith's *A compleat system of optics.*

1739   SAMUEL SHARP (1700?–1778), a prominent London surgeon, published his influential *A treatise on the operations of surgery*, which included three chapters on ophthalmology. It helped to establish extraction of cataract as opposed to couching. Sharp discusses iridectomy and iridotomy, as well as the surgical correction of lacrimal fistula.

1740   PIERRE DEMOURS (1702–1795), Parisian anatomist and ophthalmologist, gave the first report of his discoveries relating to the choroid, the cornea, and the vitreous and aqueous humors. Demours includes one of the earliest descriptions of the glass membrane of the cornea. He adds case histories regarding mydriasis and staphyloma.

1740   CLAUDE NICOLAS LE CAT (1700–1768) of Rouen published his notable work *Traité des sens*, which introduced his theory of the propagation of light contrary to that of Newtonian attraction. He also described the choroids, which he believed had a common embryonic origin with the pigmented cells of the skin. Le Cat also developed a new method for the surgical treatment of lacrimal fistula.

Pierre Demours
(1702–1795)

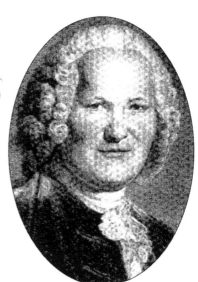

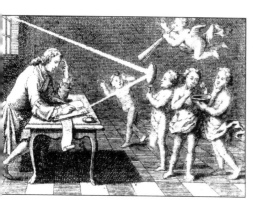

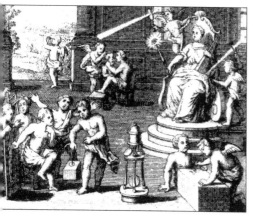

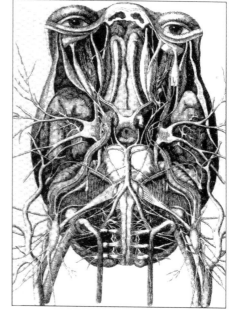

Illustrations from *Traité des sens* (1740)
by Claude Nicolas Le Cat

1742	GERALD VON SWIETEN (1706–1772) of Leiden first described the influence of belladonna on the iris in his comments on the *Aphorisms* of Hermann Boerhaave.
1743	GEORGES LOUIS LECLERC (1707–1788), the French naturalist, first suggested that poor vision could be a cause of squint, as opposed to muscular factors. Buffon claimed that in order to escape from the difficulties arising from the reception of different impressions of the same image in squint, one eye deviated.
1744	JOHN CUFF (1708?–1772) introduced brass microscopes.
1745	SIR HANS SLOANE (1660–1753), naturalist and physician, born in Ireland, published his work *An account of a most efficacious medicine for soreness, weakness, and several other distempers of the eye*. Here Sloane asserts the healing powers of an ointment consisting of the fat of vipers (which Sloane replaced with pig lard), zinc oxide, iron oxide, and aloe. Sloane claimed the ointment removed corneal scars and assuaged eye pain.
1745	JOSEPH HIGGS of Birmingham, England, published a small pamphlet that suggests treating high myopia with lens removal.
1746	JACQUES DAVIEL was appointed personal ophthalmologist to Louis XV.
1749	The French encyclopedist and philosopher, DENIS DIDEROT (1713–1784), published his controversial *Lettre sur les aveugles à la'usage de ceux qui voient*. He suggested the possibility of teaching the blind to read through the sense of touch. Diderot discussed the psychological and cognitive effects of blindness and the implication of these effects. He claimed that a blind person's moral and intellectual views vary greatly from those of sighted people. His unorthodox opinions resulted in his imprisonment for several months.
1749	DOMENICO BILLI (fl. 1750) with his work *Breve trattoto delle malatie* [sic] *degli occhi* undertook to provide specific surgical directives for the treatment of eye disease rather than leave treatment to itinerant oculists.
1750	NATALE GUISEPPE PALLUCCI (1719–1797), court surgeon in Vienna, published *Description d'un nouvel instrument pour à abaisser la cataracte*. This outlined his method of cataract depression in which he used a trocar-canula, a knife of his own invention, to cut the sclera. This enabled him to perform the depression operation without injury to the iris or ciliary body. Pallucci advocated this method instead of cataract extraction.
1750	SYLVESTER O'HALLORAN (1728–1807) of Limerick, Ireland attempted to distinguish between cataract and glaucoma in his *A new treatise on*

the glaucoma or cataract. He reviews the historical descriptions of glaucoma with the 'sky blue' pupil, which gives it its name and notes that there are no certain signs to distinguish glaucoma from cataract. O'Halloran concludes that glaucoma is 'an incurable cataract.'

1750   JACQUES DAVIEL in Paris performed the first cataract extraction on a living human eye. Daviel used a corneal incision to cut into the cataract and extract it. The incision was semicircular and close to the limbus forming a 'corneal flap.' The incision was made near the lower limbus because of the patient's tendency to roll the eye upward. He made a keratome incision and enlarged it with scissors.

1750   SAMUEL THEODOR QUELMALZ (1696–1747) of Leipzig studied ophthalmia neonatorum and theorized that the infection came from the mother's vagina and recommended washing the eyes of babies. His theory contradicted common beliefs about the disease and was generally rejected.

1751   ROBERT T. WHYTT (1714–1766) of Edinburgh published *An essay on the vital and other involuntary motions of animals.* Here he described his discovery that the response of the pupils to light is a reflex action (Whytt's reflex). He described this reflex in detail and observed that its afferent pathways lie in the optic nerve and the efferent pathways in the third cranial nerves.

1751   ROBERT MEAD (1673–1754), a fashionable London physician, advocated the use of ground up glass and sugar to grind down the opaque cornea. He based this procedure on Galen's description of superficial keratectomy. An account of his treatment of eye disease is included in his *Monita et praecepta medica.*

1752   DE LA FAYE advocated the use of a knife to open the cornea in cataract extraction as opposed to Daviel's use of scissors to make the corneal incision.

1753   JACQUES DAVIEL describes in the *Academie Royale de Chirurgie (Paris): Memoires* his procedure for extracapsular cataract extraction. His case study on his treatment had 182 successes out of 206 operations. The adoption of his surgery, over a decade later, marked the separation of ophthalmology from general surgery.

1753   SAMUEL SHARP at Guy's Hospital was the first to employ on a living patient a knife to make a corneal incision for a cataract extraction. Sharp is also credited with performing the first intracapsular cataract extraction the same year.

1754   JOSEPH WARNER (1717–1801), Samuel Sharp's student and his successor at Guy's Hospital, devised an improved cataract knife for use in Daviel's cataract extraction operation. This instrument came into wide use.

1755 BENJAMIN MARTIN established himself in London as a retailer of spectacles and scientific instruments.

1755 JACQUES DAVIEL gave a speech to the Royal Society on the importance of completely excising cancer and all affected tissues from the lids and adjacent tissues. The title of his lecture was 'A dissertation upon the cancer of the eyelids, nose, great angle of the eye, and its neighboring parts.'

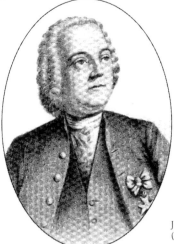

Jacques Daviel
(1696–1762)

1755 JOHANN GOTTFRIED ZINN (1727–1759), professor of medicine at Göttingen, published *Descriptio anatomica oculi humani iconibus illustrata*. This was the first complete anatomy of the eye. The descriptions of the ocular blood vessels and nerves are remarkable for their precision and thoroughness. Zinn made important discoveries concerning the iris, ciliary body, lens, and ophthalmic nerves. The

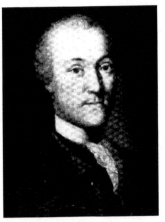

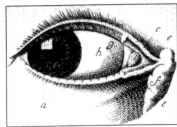

Zinn's drawing of the lacrimal system

Johann Gottfried Zinn
(1727–1759)

annulus of Zinn and zonule of Zinn are named for him.

1756   PETRUS CAMPER (1722–1789) of Leiden published *Dissertation optical de visu* together with *Dissertation physiologica de quibusdam oculi partibus.* Camper was among the first to report the lens' fibrous structure and discusses his original studies regarding the optics of the eye.

1756   MIKHAIL VASILEVICH LOMONOSOV (1711–1765) proposed that there was a separate retinal mechanism for each primary color.

1757   JACQUES RENÉ TENON (1842–1816) of Paris wrote *De cataracte,* presenting strong arguments in favor of extraction of the cataract, as opposed to couching.

1758   JEAN DESCEMET (1732–1810), a Paris ophthalmologist for whom Descemet's membrane is named, published *Quaestio medica chirurgica An sola lens crystalline caratactae sedes?* This work describes his finding of the posterior corneal 'glass' membrane. Demours contested Descemet for priority, but the membrane was actually first described by Duddell in 1729.

1758   PERCIVALL POTT (1714–1788), surgeon at St. Bartholomew's Hospital in London, published *Observations on that disorder of the corner of the eye commonly called fistula lacrimalis,* defining the methods of curing this disease.

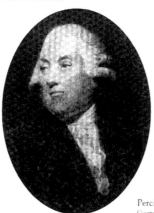

Percivall Pott (1714–1788)
Courtesy of Francis A. Countway Library of Medicine, Boston, MA

1758–1828   FRANZ JOSEPH GALL, the founder of phrenology, believed that the brain was made up of separate organs, including those concerned with sight. The individual parts were also linked with various intellectual and moral functions.

1759   BENJAMIN MARTIN produced early achromatic objectives for the microscopes.

1759   ALBRECHT VON HALLER (1708–1777), the Swiss founder of modern physiology, demonstrated that irritability or contractility is the specific property of muscular tissue, while sensibility is exclusive to nervous tissue. In his important studies of the anatomy and psychology of the visual apparatus, he extended these findings to the pupillary reflex.

1759   WILLIAM PORTERFIELD (1696–1771), a professor at the University of Edinburgh, published his two-volume work *Treatise on the eye, the manner and phenomena of vision*. Porterfield invented a simple apparatus to estimate the amplitude of accommodation and named this the 'optometer.'

1760   JOHANN HEINRICH LAMBERT (1728–1777), the founder of the science of photometry, published *Photometria*. This, together with his *Les preprietés remarquables de la route de la lumière* (1759), laid the foundation for the science of the measurement of light.

1760   ERASMUS DARWIN (1731–1802) suggested using trephination for the treatment of corneal opacity. He outlined his method in detail 'strongly recommending' it to 'some ingenious surgeon or oculist.'

1761   THOMAS GATAKER (d. 1769), surgeon to the English king, published *An account of the structure of the eye*. This was a collection of his lectures given at the Theatre of Surgeons' Hall and also discussed the use of ointments and eye-waters.

1761   GIOVANNI BATTISTA MORGAGNI (1682–1771), professor of anatomy at Padua, founded modern pathological anatomy with his monumental *De sedibus, et causis morborum per anatomen indagatis libri quinque*. Morgagni's particular significance to ophthalmology lies in his having been one of the first and most authoritative Italian proponents of the recently proposed concept of cataract as an opacification of the crystalline lens.

1762   Ophthalmology was officially recognized as a surgical subspecialty in France with the creation of the first ophthalmology chair at the École de Chirurgie in Paris by Louis XV. LOUIS FLORENT DESHAIS-GENDRON (fl. 1770) was selected as the head of the department authorized to establish a course of instruction in ophthalmology.

1765   JEAN COLOMBIER (1736–1789), a French military surgeon, published *Dissertatio nova de suffusione seu cataracta; oculi anatome & mecanismo locupletata*. One of the first proponents of cataract extraction, Colombier covered a number of aspects regarding cataract, including causes, diagnosis, and various operative procedures used.

1765   FELICE FONTANA (1730–1805), Italian naturalist and physiologist, associated the pupillary reflex with light falling on the retina. He also noted the effect of cerebral excitement upon the dilation of the pupil.

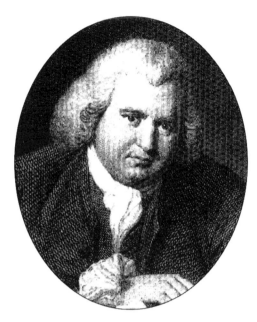

Erasmus Darwin (1731–1802)
Courtesy of Francis A. Countway
Library of Medicine, Boston, MA

Albrecht von Haller
(1708–1777)

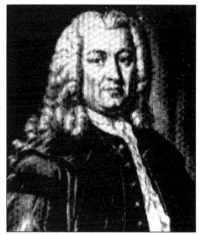

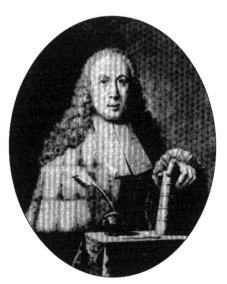

Giovanni Battista Morgagni (1682–1771)
Courtesy of Francis A. Countway Library
of Medicine, Boston, MA

1768   WILLIAM HEBERDEN (1710–1801), the distinguished London physician, reported on nyctalopia, the lack of sight at night, in a paper given to the College of Physicians of London.

1769   LEONHARD EULER (1707–1783) the Swiss mathematician, published his three-volume *Dioptricae explicatione principiorum* while on the faculty of the Academy of Sciences in St. Petersburg. It discusses the properties of lenses and the construction of dioptric instruments, particularly the microscope and telescope.

1769   PIERRE GUÉRIN (1740–1827), chief surgeon at the Hôtel Dieu in Lyons, proposed a modification of the cataract extraction operation using an instrument of his own design in his *Traité sur les maladies des yeux.*

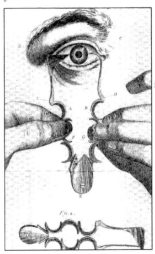

Illustration of an instrument of Guérin's own design from *Traité sur les maladies des yeux* (1769) by Pierre Guérin

1770   LOUIS FLORENT DESHAIS-GENDRON published *Traité des maladies des yeux.* It records many advances in the treatment of eye disease.

1770 – 1776   AUGUST GOTTLIEB RICHTER (1742–1812), considered the reformer of German surgery, published *Observationum chirurgicarum continens de*

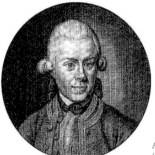

August Gottlieb Richter
(1742–1812)

cataractae extractione observations in which he advocates intracapsular cataract extraction over both couching and extracapsular cataract extraction. Richter describes his method of mobilizing the lens with a small tubule.

1771 WILLIAM ROWLEY (1743–1806) of London published his work *An essay on ophthlamia or inflammation of the eyes*. He also published a general work on eye disease in 1773, *A treatise on the principal diseases of the eyes*. Rowley issued a plagiarized translation of Plenck's *Doctrina de morbus oculorum* in 1790, which was considered in England to be an important work and was not recognized as a plagiarism for nearly half a century.

1772 JOSEPH PRIESTLEY (1733–1804), English scientist and theologist, published *History and present state of discoveries relating to vision light and colours*. Priestley, a supporter of the corpuscular theory of light, attempted to provide direct experimental proof of this hypothesis in opposition to the wave theory, but his knowledge of mathematics was inadequate for the task.

1772 JEAN JANIN (1731–1799), ophthalmic surgeon in Lyon, published *Memoir et observations sur l'oeil* that described the use of convex lenses to see distant objects. He operated with great skill and published valuable observations on cataract, the lacrimal apparatus, and binocular vision.

1773 Empress Maria Theresa appointed JOSEPH BARTH (1745–1818), professor of ophthalmology and anatomy at the University of Vienna, the 'Lecturer on Eye Diseases'. Barth's first pupils were Johann Adam Schmidt and Georg Joseph Beer. This was followed by his appointment as oculist to Emperor Joseph II in 1776.

1775 The existence of an annular canal through which aqueous exits the eye (i.e. canal of Schlemm) was illustrated and described in a catalogue of preparations from the late BERNHARD SIEGFRIED ALBINUS (1697–1770), professor of anatomy and surgery at Leiden. Albinus termed this *sinus venosus*. He was also the first to provide a depiction of congenital coloboma of the iris and helped clarify the origin of the optic nerves.

1775 CHRISTIAN KÄSTNER described the optics of hypermetropia, expanding on Hambruger's earlier explanation.

1775 JOHAN LORENZ ODHELIUS (1737–) of Sweden gave his lecture entitled 'Anmärkingar vid starr-operationen och den sjukes skotsel derefter' to the Royal Academy of Science in Stockholm. The speech was his cataract extraction method based on that of Jacques Daviel, and was responsible for popularizing Daviel's technique.

1775	PERCIVALL POTT of St. Bartholomew's Hospital in London in his *Surgical Observations* opposed cataract extraction. He suggests discussion as a regular means of treatment for soft cataract.
1777	JOSEPH JACOB RITTER VON PLENCK (1738–1807) of Vienna authored *Doctrina de morbis oculorum* on his lecture series of eye disease. It was among the last of the popular ophthalmic textbooks to be published in Latin.
1777	A surgeon named SIMON in Paris gave public demonstrations of cataract extraction. These were witnessed by Christian Gotthold Keller (1755–1785), a medical student at Leipzig, who described the procedure in 1782.
1777	JOSEPH PRIESTLEY reported an early case of color blindness communicated to him by William Huddart. The patient, a man named Harris, realized that he could not discern colors and that he shared the affliction with his two brothers.
1778	SAMUEL THOMAS VON SOEMMERRING (1755–1830) published his doctoral dissertation at the University of Göttingen, presenting the classification of the cranial nerves that is still taught.

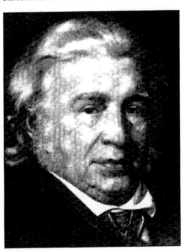

Samuel Thomas von Soemmerring
(1755–1830)

| 1779 | The techniques and instruments employed by the famous German itinerant cataract extractor MICHAEL VON WENZEL (d. 1790) are described by his son and pupil JACOB DE WENZEL (1755–1810) in his doctoral dissertation *De extractione cataractae*. |
| 1779 | CASAAMATA (fl. 1779–1806), an Italian-born itinerant cataract surgeon and later Dresden court-ophthalmologist, made a false claim of curing strabismus with a very small segatura. |

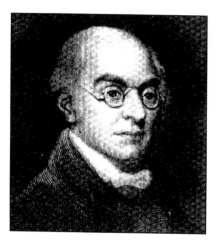

Joseph Ware
(1756–1815)

1780   JAMES WARE (1756–1815), a London ophthalmologist, recognized the mode of transmission of venereal ophthalmia in the adult but states that infection in the newborn arises from a cold. In his *Remarks on the ophthalmy, psorophthalmy and purulent eye*, he recommends repeated and regular irrigation with copper sulfate for venereal ophthalmia.

1780   JOSEPH JAKOB VON MOHRENHEIM (ca. 1759–1799), ophthalmologist, surgeon, and obstetrician, published *Beobachtungen verschiedener chirurgischer Vorfälle*. The author, a skilled cataract surgeon, reports on his experiences with the extraction operation but concludes that he still prefers couching for cataract.

1780   MICHELE TROJA (1747–1827) of Italy published his work on ophthalmology entitled *Lezioni intorno alle malattie degli occhi*. He discusses his technique for creating artificial cataracts in cadavers' eyes on which beginners can practice surgical techniques.

1780   JEAN PAUL MARAT (1743–1793), a major figure in the French Revolution, published *Découvertes sur la lumière*. This, combined with his *Notions élémentaires d'optique*, contradicted Newton's theory of light emissions. Marat developed his own theories of colors and light, which were based on more than 200 experiments.

1781   JONATHAN WATHEN (1729–1808), a surgeon and ophthalmologist in London, published *A new and easy method of applying a tube for the cure of the fistula lachrymalis*. This includes maintaining the patency of the nasolacrimal duct by inserting a gold tubule of his own design.

1781   FELICE FONTANA in his *Traité sur vénim de la vipere* (1781) included a letter to 'Mr. Adolphe Murray, celebrated professor of anatomy at Uppsala' on pages 267–69 wherein he describes his discovery of a new canal that exists in herbivores. The term Fontana's space is still used for the intertrabecular spaces of the human corneoscleral meshwork, although it is not analogous to the structure Fontana described.

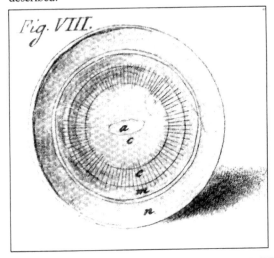

Illustration of the 'canal of Fontana' from *Traité sur vénim de la vipere* (1781) by Felice Fontana

1782	CHRISTIAN GOTTLIEB FELLER, physician to Bautzen, Germany, published *De methodis suffusione oculorum curandi*. This documented the cataract extractions of Simon in Paris (1777) and Casa Amata in Leipzig (1779) and exists as the only record of their procedures.

1782   FRANCESCO BUZZI (1751–1805), ophthalmic surgeon at the Speciale Mattiori in Milan, was the first to describe the macula lutea of the human retina.

1782   PAOLO ASSALINI (1759–1840), an Italian surgeon, was among the first to use iridodialysis to produce an artificial pupil.

1783   ALEXANDER MONRO, *secundus* (1733–1817), professor of anatomy and surgery at the University of Edinburgh, published *Observations on the structure and functions of the nervous system* in which he described the foramen interventriculare (foramen of Monro).

1783   WILLIAM BUTTER (1726–1805), an ophthalmologist in London and Derby, published *An improved method of opening the temporal artery. Also, a new proposal for extracting the cataract*. Chapter 4 discusses cataract extraction and proposes that this procedure replace depression of the cataract. He describes in detail his method of extraction and the instrument to be employed.

1783   ANDRE BOSCHE in a thesis at Montpellier described a procedure for closure of the canaliculi through chemical destruction.

1783   GUILLAUME PELLIER DE QUENGSY (1850/51?–1855), distinguished ophthalmic surgeon of Montpellier, describes in his *Recueil de mémoires* a new instrument, the 'ophthalmotome,' which enabled him to perform cataract extraction with one swift maneuver.

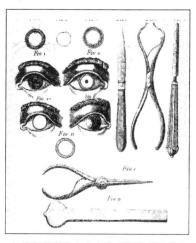

Illustration from *Precis ou cours d'operations sur la chirurgie* (1789) by Pellier de Quengsy

1784   GIOVANNI AMBROGIO MARIA BERTRANDI (1723–1765), a professor of ophthalmology in Turin, published *Traité des opérations de chirurgie*. Several chapters discuss ophthalmic surgery.

1784   VALENTIN HAÜY (1745–1822), educator of the blind, established the Institution des Jeunes Aveugles in Saint-Just, France, the first school for the blind. Haüy was the first to make texts with raised characters available to the blind, and developed courses of instruction for blind children. Haüy went on to aid with the establishment of similar schools in Russia and Germany.

1784   BENJAMIN FRANKLIN (1706–1790) made mention of bifocals in a letter to his colleague, George Whatley. He is commonly credited with their

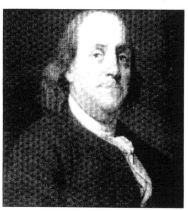

Benjamin Franklin (1706–1790)

59

invention, and bifocals quickly became popular.

1784   ANTOINE PIERRE DEMOURS (1762–1836), famed French ophthalmologist and son of Pierre Demours, stressed the importance of mydriasis as a preliminary procedure in various ophthalmic operations.

1785   JONATHAN WATHEN of London published A *dissertation on the theory and care of cataract.* He mentions his controversial support of the extraction procedure against the opposition of influential English surgeons. He offers details about his own techniques and instruments.

1785   VON WILLBURG proposed replacing the usual couching procedure by a method of couching that displaced the lens backward, called reclination. Scarpa, Dupuytren, and Christophe Lusardi advocated this method.

1786   JUSTUS ARNEMANN, professor at Göttingen, published *Übersicht der Berühmtesten und Gevrauchlichsten Chirurgischen Instrumente* in which he, like George Joseph Beer, advocated intracapsular extraction for cataracts.

1786   JEAN FRANÇOIS GLEIZE (fl. 1763–1811), oculist to the Duke of Orléans, published *Nouvelles observations pratiques sur les maladies de l'oeil.* An advocate and successful practitioner of cataract extraction, he directed his book to the public.

1786   JOHN HUNTER (1728–1793), a renowned biologist, researcher, and surgeon, published *Observations on certain parts of the animal oeconomy,* which contains one of the earliest descriptions of the ocular pigment epithelium. He also published important studies on the ophthalmic effects of venereal disease.

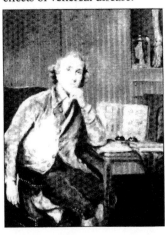

John Hunter (1728–1793)

1786   The first known eye hospital was founded in Vienna by GEORG JOSEPH BEER (1763–1821). He became the most celebrated ophthalmic surgeon of his day and founded the Vienna School of Ophthalmology. Beer pioneered the iridectomy, accurately described the symptoms of acute glaucoma, and described the luminosity of the fundus in cases of aniridia. More than any other person, Beer was responsible for the development of ophthalmology as an independent medical and surgical specialty in Europe.

1786   SAMUEL THOMAS VON SOEMMERRING demonstrated the crossing of the optic nerve fibers.

1786   L'ABBÉ DESMONCEAUX (1734–1806), a priest and physician, published *Traité des maladies des yeux et des oreilles* advocating extraction of the clear lens for treatment of high myopia.

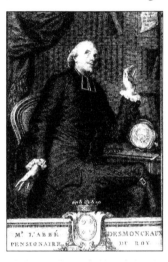

Frontispiece from *Traité des maladies des yeux et des oreilles* (1786) by L'Abbé Desmonceaux

1787   PAOLO ASSALINI, an Italian surgeon, reported that when trying to extract an opaque adherent lens capsule with a forceps through a corneal incision, he tore one-third of the iris from its root. This resulted in a useful new pupil.

1788   FRANCESCO BUZZI of Milan was among the early surgeons to intentionally create a new pupil by iridodialysis.

1789   GUILLAUME PELLIER DE QUENGSY of Montpellier described the first keratoprosthesis in his ophthalmic text *Precis ou cours d'operations sur la chirurgie*. This constitutes one of the earliest attempts to treat scarred corneas surgically. Pellier de Quengsy's method consisted of making an artificial cornea out of glass and substituting it for the scarred cornea of the patient. He includes his technique for cataract extraction, diseases of the vitreous, cases requiring removal of the eye, and a discussion of diseases of the lid and lacrimal sac.

1791 The Edinburgh Asylum, to serve the blind, was established by EDWARD RUSHTON and J. CHRISTIE, who were both blind.

1791 JOHANN ADAM SCHMIDT (1759–1809) founded an eye infirmary in Vienna.

1791 SAMUEL THOMAS VON SOEMMERRING discovered the fovea centralis (macula flava) in the macula lutea. He believed this to be an actual perforation in the retina, which was responsible for the 'blind spot of Mariotte' in the field of vision.

1792 WILLIAM CHARLES WELLS (1757–1817), an American Royalist, published *An essay upon single vision with two eyes: together with experiments and observations on several other subjects in optics.* Wells wrote two other essays on the physiology of vision (1810, 1811), and all three discuss fusion, accommodation, and hypermetropia.

1792 GEORG JOSEPH BEER published *Lehre der Augenkrankheiten.* He described the symptoms of glaucoma and noted the luminosity of the fundus in aniridia. In the same year, he recorded the first known case of tobacco amblyopia.

1793 JOAQUIM JOSÉ DE SANTA ANNA, ophthalmologist at the Royal Hospital at San José, Portugal, published *Elementos de cirurgia ocular.* This was intended to update and expand *Doctrina de morbis oculorum* (1777) by Joseph Jacob Plenck of Vienna.

1793 THOMAS YOUNG (1773–1829), English physician, physicist, and Egyptologist, demonstrated that accommodation of the eye is due to change of curvature in the crystalline lens in his paper 'Observations on vision.' He theorizes that the lens is composed of muscle fibers that, by contracting, make the lens more convex.

1794 THOMAS PERCIVAL (1740–1804) of Manchester, England privately published *Medical ethics.* The recommendations it included comprise the foundation of modern medical ethics in England, America, and other countries. It was formally published in 1803.

1794 MATTHEW BAILLIE (1761–1823) published *The morbid anatomy of some of the most important parts of the human body.* It served as a model for JAMES WARDROP'S *Essays on the morbid anatomy of the human eye* (1808), the first ophthalmic pathology text.

1795 CASAAMATA in Dresden was probably the first to attempt to surgically treat aphakia with intraocular lenses. He inserted crystal spheres into the pupil through the wound in the cornea, but noted that the glass lens fell to the bottom of the eye. He took this idea from Giacomo Casanova (1725–1798), who in turn

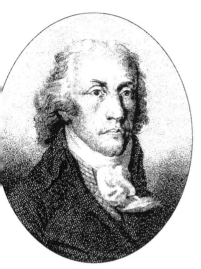

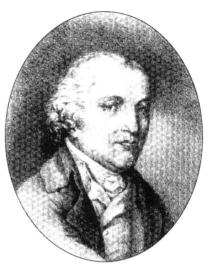

ohann Adam Schmidt (1759–1809)
rtesy of Francis A. Countway Library of
Medicine, Boston, MA

Georg Joseph Beer (1763–1821)
Courtesy of Francis A. Countway
Library of Medicine, Boston, MA

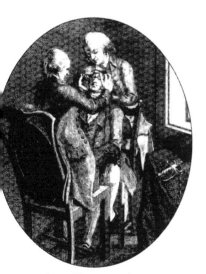

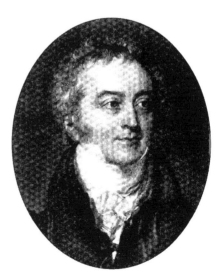

stration from *Elementos de cirurgia ocular*
793) by Joaquim José de Santa Anna

Thomas Young
(1773–1829)

had learned of it from Tadini, an oculist.

1795   JAMES WARE, a London ophthalmologist, recognized and described the venereal nature of ophthalmia neonatorum in his *Additional remarks on the ophthalmy*.

1796   The *Y'en K'e Ta CH'eng* (*Great success of ophthalmology*), (also *Yen hai chih nan*, or *Compass of the silver sea*) was published by YANG WU. In it the eye is compared to the sea, and the book to a compass to guide physicians. The second volume discusses the relationship between ocular diseases and other diseases, and connects ocular diseases with specific organs.

1796   JESSE RAMSDEN (1735–1800) invented the keratometer to detect any change in corneal curvature. Helmholtz in 1854 designed a keratometer to determine the radius of curvature of the anterior corneal surface.

1797   JOSEPH BARTH of Vienna published *Etwas über die Ausziehung des grauen Staares*. In it he gives instructions on the extraction of the cataract.

1798   JOHN DALTON (1766–1844), the English scientist and teacher himself afflicted with red–green blindness, gave the first scientific description of this defect in his *Extraordinary facts relating to the vision of colours*. Dalton attributed this fault to a blue pigment in the vitreous humor. This condition has subsequently been called 'Daltonism.'

1798   GEORG JOSEPH BEER of Vienna described his method of iridectomy, a procedure in which he made an artificial pupil by removing part of the iris. Beer devised a special blade to perform this procedure.

1799   BENJAMIN GIBSON (1774–1812) of England, student of Braille, settled in Manchester to practice medicine.

1800   KARL HIMLY (1772–1837) of Göttingen was the rediscoverer of artificial mydriusis and made the first use of hyoscyamus surgery for pupil dilation in cataract. He popularized the employment of mydriatics prior to and following eye surgery and provided the first accurate and systematic discussion of their effects.

1801   SIR JAMES EARLE (1755–1817), surgeon at St. Bartholomew's Hospital and surgeon extraordinary to George III, published *An account of a new mode of operation for the removal of the opacity in the eye, called cataract*. He describes his new technique for cataract extraction surgery.

1801   JOHANN ADAM SCHMIDT of Vienna published *Über Nachstaar und Iritis nach Staaroperation* dealing with after-cataract and inflammation of the iris following cataract surgery. Schmidt favored extracapsular cataract extraction over the intracapsular technique advocated by Beer.

1801   THOMAS YOUNG of London gave the first description of astigmatism. Also in 1801, Young first stated the theory that color vision is due to retinal structures corresponding with red, green, and violet.

1801   ANTONIO SCARPA (1752–1832), one of the greatest anatomists and surgeons of all time, wrote his classic ophthalmologic text *Saggio di osservazzioni e d'esperience sulle principali malattie degli occhi*. It includes a description of Scarpa's iridodialysis procedure for the creation of an artificial pupil.

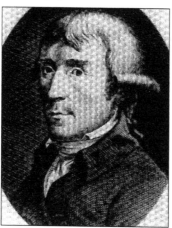

Antonio Scarpa
(1752–1832)

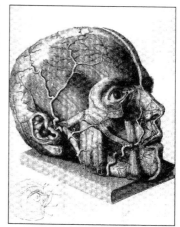

Illustration from *Saggio di osservazzioni e d'esperience sulle principali malattie degli occhi* (1801) by Antonio Scarpa

1801   *Ophthalmologische Bibliothek*, the first ophthalmic journal, was established by KARL HIMLY of Göttingen and JOHANN ADAM SCHMIDT of Vienna. This journal continued to be published until 1807.

1801–1803   THOMAS YOUNG of London advanced his wave theory of light.

1801   GERARDUS VROLIK (1775–1859), an anatomist and surgeon at the Athenaeum Illustre of Amsterdam, showed that the crystalline lens could proliferate after extracapsular cataract surgery. He gave the first exact description of a Soemmerring's ring cataract.

1802–1833   SIR CHARLES BELL (1774–1842) and FRANÇOIS MAGENDIE (1783–1855) independently studied and described the role of the spinal cord's anterior and posterior roots. The posterior roots carry information from the sensory organs, while the anterior roots are motor nerves. This information came to be referred to as the Bell–Magendie law.

1801   DOMINIQUE JEAN LARREY (1766–1842), surgeon-in-chief to Napoleon's Grande Armée, was the first to point out the contagious nature of Egyptian ophthalmia (trachoma) in his *Mémoire sur l'ophtalmie regnente en Egypte*.

1803   JOHANN ADAM SCHMIDT published *Über Krankeiten des Thränenorgans*, the first extensive monograph devoted entirely to diseases of the lacrimal system.

1804   WILLIAM HYDE WOLLASTON (1766–1828) patented his 'periscope spectacles.' These substituted meniscus lenses for the generally used biconvex and biconcave forms to allow clear sight in oblique directions for those with astigmatism.

1804   SAMUEL THOMAS SOEMMERRING of Münich published *Abildungen des menschlichen Auges*. This beautiful anatomical atlas shows front and profile views of diagrams of the living eyes of whites and blacks, as well as an albino.

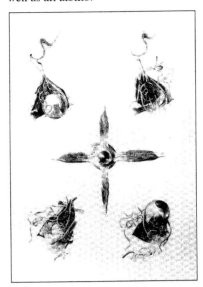

Illustration of the eye from Soemmerring's series of illustrations of the human sense organs (1801–1809) from *Abildungen des menschlichen Auges* (1804)

1804   DIETRICH GEORG KIESER (1779–1862), who directed an ophthalmologic clinic in Jena, proved that Fontana's space, which was described in herbivores in 1765, was not part of the human ocular anatomy.

1805   WILLIAM HEY (1736–1819), a senior surgeon at Leeds Infirmary, published *Practical observations in surgery*. This includes a section on cataract and an early description of retinoblastoma, then called fungus haematodes.

1805   JOHN CUNNINGHAM SAUNDERS (1773–1810) founded Moorfields Eye Hospital. Originally named the London Dispensary for Curing Diseases of the Eye and Ears, and later the Royal London Ophthalmic Hospital, this institution attempted to deal with the epidemic of Egyptian ophthalmia brought to England by the return of infected sailors and soldiers from the Napoleonic Wars. Saunders remained its director until his death five years later. Other eye institutions in the United Kingdom and America were modeled after Moorfields.

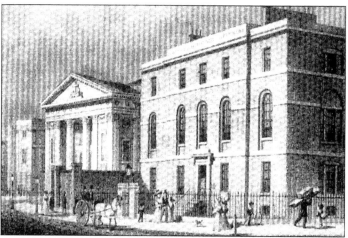

Moorfields Eye Hospital, London

1805   JAMES WARE described the pathologic appearance of a retinal detachment.

1805   JACQUES RENÉ TENON, a Parisian anatomist and surgeon, first described the fibrous capsule (Tenon's capsule) that covers much of the globe. The paper was published the next year in his *Mémoirs et observations sur l'anatomie, la pathologie et la chirurgie*. Tenon explains the relationship of this capsule to the ocular muscles. Modern enucleation became possible when surgeons understood the nature of Tenon's capsule.

1806   ARTHUR EDMONDSTON (1776?–1841), an army surgeon in Egypt who later practiced medicine in the Shetland Islands, published *A treatise on the varieties and consequences of ophthalmia*. Edmonston was one of the first to demonstrate the contagious nature of the disease.

1806   WILHELM HEINRICH BUCHHORN devised a new cataract operation called keratonyxis. A special rounded needle is used to perforate the cornea and incise the lens capsule. This approach could also be used to fragment the cataract.

1806   ANTONIO SCARPA in Pavia carried out what appears to be the first documented ptosis procedure. He excised integuments at the upper part of the relaxed eyelid in the vicinity and direction of the superior arch of the orbit.

1807   JOHN VETCH (1783–1835), a medical officer in the British army, published *An account of the ophthalmia, which has appeared in England since the return of the British Army from Egypt*. He gives a history of trachoma in the British army, describes its symptoms, and details the various treatments that have been tried. Vetch is the first to assert that the means of infection is exclusively through transmission of exudates from a diseased eye to a healthy eye.

1807   THOMAS YOUNG of London published *Lecture on optical instruments*. Here Young provides the principal explanation of astigmatism produced by oblique refraction of rays through spherical lenses. He demonstrates that 'the effect of obliquity of the different pencils of rays materially increases the curvature of the image.' Young notes that a curved receiving surface—such as the retina—is necessary for a sharp image.

1808   JACOB DE WENZEL of Paris, ophthalmologist to the Imperial family, published *Manuel de l'oculiste, our dictionnaire ophthalmologique*. This was the first handbook of ophthalmology to be arranged as a dictionary.

1808   LEOPOLDO CALDANI (1725–1813), anatomist and physiologist at Padua, confirmed Haller's findings and theories regarding the papillary reflex in his *Intorno ai movimenti dell'iride dell'occhio*.

1808   The first volume of JAMES WARDROP'S (1782–1869) *Morbid anatomy of the human eye* was published, dealing primarily with the cornea. Wardrop was the founder of ophthalmic pathology. He was the first to organize ophthalmic inflammation according to the structure affected. In this work Wardrop introduces the term 'keratitis.'

1809   JAMES WARDROP published *Observations on the fungus haematodes*,

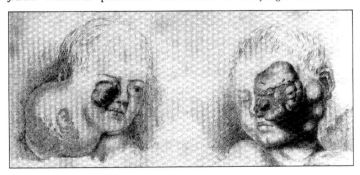

Illustration from *Observations on the fungus haematodes* (1809) by James Wardrop

establishing retinoblastoma as a specific type of cancer. Wardrop advocated enucleation as the best treatment.

1809   THOMAS YOUNG demonstrated the application of the wave theory of light to crystalline refraction and dispersion phenomena.

1809   CARLO DONEGANA (1776–1828) of Como, published his improvement of Scarpa's iridodialysis procedure in *Della pupilla artificiale*. He used a special needle to detach the iris and then incised it from its circumference toward its center.

1810   JEAN LOUIS PRÉVOST (1790–1850) of Geneva demonstrated that the luminosity of animal pupils is merely a reflection of light.

1810   JOHN STEVENSON (1778–1846), a London ophthalmologist and surgeon, established a cataract clinic that he called 'Dispensary for Cataractous Patients.' The name was later changed to 'Ophthalmic Institute for the Cure of Cataract' (1823). Stevenson preferred the discission procedure employed by Saunders and added some modifications of his own.

1810   JOHANN WOLFGANG GOETHE (1749–1832), German poet, dramatist, novelist, and scientist, published his theory of color, *Zur Farbenlehre*. This theory was based on his experiments with prisms from which he concluded that all colors are darker than white, and they have something of shade in them. Goethe maintained that colors owe their existence to some form of cooperation between light and shadow. He insisted that the eye took an active, rather than passive, role in the act of seeing. Goethe attacked Newton's theory that white light is a composite of color.

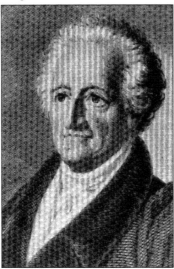

Johann Wolfgang Goethe
(1749–1832)

1810   JEAN GABRIEL AUGUST CHEVALLIER (1778–1848), a French optician and instrument maker, published *Le conservateur de la vue, suivi du catalogue général et prix courant des instrumens d'optique*. It discusses the ocular anatomy of the eye and describes eyeglasses, binoculars, telescopes, and microscopes. Also included is a catalogue of spectacles and instruments available for sale by the Chevallier firm. Chevallier invented a great variety of optical instruments, perfected others, and devised some of the earliest vision tests, involving the reading of print.

1810   TRAUGOTT WILHELM GUSTAV BENEDICT (1785–1862), a prominent Breslau ophthalmologist, published *De pupillae artificialis conformatione libellus*. He describes multiple types of artificial pupil surgery, including iridotomy, iridectomy, and iridodialysis.

1810   BENEDICT PREVOST (1755–1819) in Montauben, France repeated Edme Mariotte's experiments examining the eyes of a cat in the dark and confirmed that reflected light is the only source of the luminosity of the eyes of animals.

1811   SÉBASTIAN GUILLIÉ (1780–1865), French ophthalmologist and teacher of the blind, replaces Valentin Haüy as director of the Institution des Jeunes Aveugles in Paris. Louis Braille was Guillié's student.

1811   PAOLO ASSALINI, now Napoleon's surgeon and professor in Milan, published *Ricerche sulle pupille artificiali*. In this monograph on artificial pupils, he evaluated the various procedures for the formation of a new pupil. Assalini also modifyied Pellier's lid retractor and Scarpa's needle for cataracts.

1812   GILBERT ALPHONSE CLAUDE MONTAIN (1780–1853), chief surgeon at the Charité in Lyons, published *Traité de la cataracte* in which he describes several ophthalmic instruments he invented for the depression of cataracts, including a spring instrument. Montain became eminent as a depressor of cataracts.

1812   JEAN PIERRE MAUNOIR (1768–1861), anatomy professor at the Académie Impériale in Geneva, published *Mémoires sur l'organisation de l'iris et l'opération de la pupille artificielle*. This described his iridectomy technique, which was widely adopted by ophthalmic surgeons.

1812   WILLIAM ADAMS (1783–1827), a London ophthalmologist, proposed tarsal wedge resection to treat ectropion, using a narrow knife of his own design. The operation was similar to that of Antyllus of the second century AD and is described in his *Practical observations on ectropion*.

1813   THOMAS JOHANN SEEBECK (1770–1831) of Jena discovered the entopic color phenomena.

1813   DAVID HOSACK (1769–1835), professor of medicine at the College of Physicians in New York City, published *Observations on vision*, which included his studies on accommodation.

1813   SIR DAVID BREWSTER (1781–1868) of Edinburgh published *A treatise on new philosophical instruments with experiments on light and colours.* Brewster described his experiments on light and colors. He coined the term 'color blindness.' He produced the kaleidoscope and the lenticular stereoscope and described telescopes, micrometers, and the catadioptric microscope.

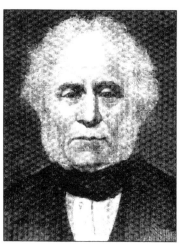

Sir David Brewster (1781–1868)
Courtesy of Francis A. Countway Library of Medicine, Boston, MA

1813   JOHN SYNG DORSEY (1783–1818) of Philadelphia published the teachings of his uncle PHILLIP SYNG PHYSICK (1768–1837), professor of anatomy and surgery at the University of Pennsylvania, *Elements of surgery*. It includes chapters on ophthalmic diseases and surgery for cataracts. Physick began his surgical practice in 1792 and became a notable eye surgeon. He invented a punch used for the formation of an artificial pupil.

1813   FRANÇOIS MAGENDIE, the French pioneer in experimental physiology, demonstrated the formation of retinal images by removing the fat from around the eye of a freshly killed albino rabbit and holding the eye to the light so that the images of external objects could be seen through the thin sclera at the back of the eyeball. This is described in his paper *Mémoire sur les images qui se forment au fond de l'oeil*.

1814   TRAUGOTT WILHELM BENEDICT of Breslau discovered the etiologic relationship between cataracts and diabetes. This finding was contested by most of his contemporaries, including von Graefe. In his *Monographie der granen Staares*, he also discusses the diagnosis, etiology, and treatment of cataracts generally.

1814   JOHAN HEINRICH FERDINAND AUTENRIETH (1772–1835) invented sclerectomy and described its use in *De pupilla artificiali in sclerotica apienrienda*. He conceived the idea when he saw a patient who became blind with bilateral staphylomas after an attack of smallpox. Autenrieth practiced the operation on cats' eyes, excising sclera, choroids, and retina at their anterior aspect. The defect was covered with conjunctiva, which, according to Autenrieth, appeared relatively transparent.

1814   FRANZ REISINGER (1787–1855), an ophthalmologist and surgeon in Augsburg, published *Berträge zur Chirugie und Augenheilkinde*. It includes the construction and use of an instrument for teaching purposes in ophthalmology, which is illustrated by a copper plate.

1814   WILLIAM ADAMS was awarded a knighthood for his controversial claims of curing the Egyptian ophthalmia (trachoma). Although he implied he had a new treatment, he in fact resected granulations and applied a strong copper sulfate solution. Adams became the center of controversy, and in 1817 there was a parliamentary debate on the matter.

1814   PHILIBERT JOSEPH ROUX (1780–1854), of the Hôtel Dieu in Paris, published *Memoire et observations*. Roux was a pioneer in plastic surgery and discussed his reparative surgery technique. He also gave an account of strabismus in his own right eye, which he claimed to have healed by exercises.

1814–1826   ALEXIS BOYER (1757–1833) of Paris authored a popular eleven-volume work on general surgery that devoted one volume to eyes, promoting cataract extractions.

1815–1828   KONRAD JOHANN MARTIN LANGENBECK (1775–1851), professor of anatomy and surgery in Göttingen, published *Neue Bibliothek für die Chirurgie und Ophthalmologie*. Langenbeck, a surgeon of phenomenal swiftness and dexterity, gave considerable attention to ophthalmic surgery.

c. 1815   GIOVANNI BATTISTA AMICI (1786–1863) constructed an optical system using aplanatic and achromatic lenses.

1815   GIOVANNI BATTISTA QUADRI (1780–1851), an ophthalmologist in Naples, established one of the first ophthalmic hospitals in Italy. Between 1818 and 1830, he published detailed accounts of his work in the hospital.

1816   ARTHUR SCHOPENHAUER (1788–1860), the German philosopher, at the urging of Goethe, studied the nature of colors and color vision. In

1816, he published *Über das Sehn und die Farben*. Schopenhauer concentrated on the effect of light on the retina. He believed the excitation of the retina varied depending on which color was being perceived. That is, colors varied in their ability to stimulate retinal activity.

1816   JOSEPH CONSTANTINE CARPUE (1764–1846), a distinguished English surgeon, ushered in the era of modern plastic surgery with his *An account of two successful operations for restoring a lost nose from the integuments of the forehead*. His report included descriptions of modern flap reconstruction and electrotherapy as a remedy for ocular diseases.

1816   The Westminster Ophthalmic Hospital in London was founded by GEORGE JAMES GUTHRIE (1785–1856), a famous military surgeon who excelled at ophthalmic plastic surgery. Guthrie served as the chief surgeon at the Westminster Ophthalmic Hospital until 1838.

1816   The eye infirmary in St. Petersburg was established with seventeen beds under the direction of Wilhelm Lerche (b. 1791). An ambulatory service was added in 1816.

1817   SÉBASTIEN GUILLIÉ of Paris published *Essai sur l'instruction des aveugles* in which he recorded his techniques for teaching the blind. The book was a result of his experience as director of the Institution des Jeunes Aveugles (1811).

1817   CARL HEINRICH DZONDI (1770–1835) performed eyelid reconstruction and tested new techniques of blepharoplasty. Dzondi was professor of surgery at Halle, Germany. His methods are summarized in detail in his *Die Augenheilkunde für Jedermann* (1835).

1817   ELISHA NORTH (1771–1843), who attended the University of Pennsylvania and was a pioneer vaccinator, established an eye clinic in New London, Connecticut, the first eye clinic in the United States. North was also the author of the first treatise on epidemic cerebrospinal meningitis.

1818   EDWARD REYNOLDS (1793–1881) of Boston, co-founder of the Massachusetts Eye and Ear Infirmary, performed an early cataract procedure in New England, couching both of his father's lenses in one sitting.

1818   DETMAR WILHELM SOEMMERRING (1793–1871) published his Göttingen doctoral dissertation *De oculorum hominis animaliumque sectione horizontali commentatio*. This was one of the first studies of the comparative anatomy of the eye.

1818   JULES GERMAIN CLOQUET (1790–1883), professor at the Medical

Faculty of Paris and consulting surgeon to the emperor, made important contributions to eye anatomy, starting with his 1818 publication of *Mémoire sur la membrane pupillaire, et sur la formation du petit cercle artériel de l'iris* in which the pupillary membrane was meticulously analyzed.

1818   JAMES WARDROP'S second volume of the *Morbid anatomy of the human eye* was published. This volume dealt with the iris, sclera, and ocular structures. Wardrop followed the tissue-pathology concept laid out by Bichet in his revolutionary *Anatomie générale* of 1802.

1818   FRANZ REISINGER of Augsburg suggested that one could replace a completely opaque cornea by some transparent medium.

1818   ANTOINE PIERRE DEMOURS of Paris published *Traité des maladies des yeux*, containing hundreds of case histories drawn from his and his father's (Pierre Demour's) practices. It contained one of the earliest complete descriptions of glaucoma to that time, including recognition of elevated intraocular pressure.

1818   HEINRICH CHRISTIAN BÜNGER (1782–1842), a professor of anatomy at Marburg, reported on the first verified clinically successful free-skin autograft harvested from the upper thigh and used in a case of nasal reconstruction.

1818   WILLIAM GIBSON (1788–1868), a surgeon at the University of Pennsylvania, corrected strabismus by severing the insertion of an ocular muscle. Gibson also invented scissors for cataract surgery and the 'seton method' for cataract. His contributions are described in his *Institutes and practice of surgery*.

1819   CARL HEINRICH WELLER (1794–1854), an ophthalmologist in Dresden, published *Die Kronkheiten des menschlichen Auges*. The first edition contains little original material and draws heavily on Beer's textbooks. With each subsequent edition, however, Weller added more of his own observations and reported on the latest advances in the field. The fourth and last edition appeared in 1830.

1819   HEINRICH BRUNO SCHINDLER (1834–1898) of Breslau, in *Commentatio ophthalmiatrica* (1819) and subsequent papers, discusses the various types of keratitis and gives an early description of interstitial keratitis.

1819   FRANCESCO FLARER (1791–1859) became professor of ophthalmology at Pavia. Flarer made many contributions to the treatment of cataract, iritis, and trichiasis.

1819   JAMES WARDROP of London published *An essay on the diseases of the eye of the horse and their treatment*. Wardrop recognized and accurately described sympathetic ophthalmia in humans but confuses periodic

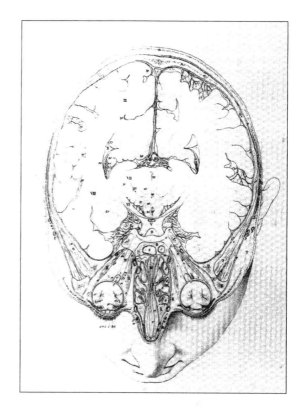

Copperplate illustration from *De oculorum hominis animaliumque sectione horizontali commentatio* (1818) by Detmar Wilhelm Soemmerring

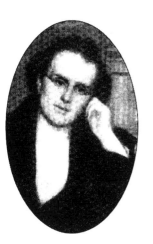

Arthur Jacob
(1790–1874)

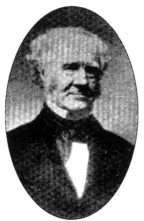

Edward Reynolds
(1793–1881)

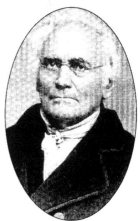

Jan Evangelista Purkinje
(1787–1869)

ophthalmia in horses with this entity.

1819   ARTHUR JACOB (1790–1874), a professor of anatomy and physiology at the Royal College of Surgeons in Dublin, discovered the layer of rods and cones in the retina. This became known as 'Jacob's membrane.'

1819   JAN EVANGELISTA PURKINJE (1787–1869), Czech pioneer in histology and physiology, published *Beitrage zur Kenntniss des Sehens in subjective Hinsicht* describing the subjective visual phenomena.

1820   JOHN VETCH of London published an experiment in which pus from the purulent conjunctivitis of a man was transferred to the urethra of another man. This caused a severe inflammation of the urethra within 36 hours.

1820   NICHOLAS JEAN FAURE (b. 1782), quack-oculist, published *Observations sur l'iris* in which he claims to have invented the already well-established cataract procedure known as discission of the lens.

1820   BENJAMIN TRAVERS (1783–1858) published *A synopsis of the diseases of the eye and their treatment*. This was the first comprehensive and systematic treatise on eye diseases published in English. Travers's book became the authoritative textbook in England and America.

1820   SEBASTIAN GUILLIÉ of Paris founded the first French journal of ophthalmology, *Bibliotheque ophtalmologique*, which was discontinued in 1822.

1820   *Journal für Chirurgie und Augenheilkunde* was founded by CARL FERDINAND VON GRAEFE (1787–1840) of Berlin and PHILIPP VON WALTHER (1782–1849) of Bonn. This became an important forum for new developments in ophthalmology.

1820   JEAN PIERRE MAUNOIR of Geneva published *Mémoire sur les fongus médulaire et hématode*, an important monograph on retinoblastoma.

1821–1831   JULES GERMAIN CLOQUET published *Anatomie de l'homme*. It was a five-volume anatomical atlas that was the earliest to use lithographs. He gave the first anatomical account of the canal of Cloquet, or the hyaloidian canal, and the role of the canal during fetal life.

1821–1822   GEORG LEBRECHT ANDREAS HELLING (1763–1840) of Berlin published *Praktisches Handbuch der Augenkrankheiten*. He invented several ophthalmic plastic procedures and a number of ophthalmic instruments.

1821   SIR ASTLEY PASTON COOPER (1768–1841), a popular and distinguished surgeon at Guy's and St. Thomas' Hospitals, published *Surgical essays, part I & II*. Of ophthalmic interest is a chapter on iritis contributed by Benjamin Travers.

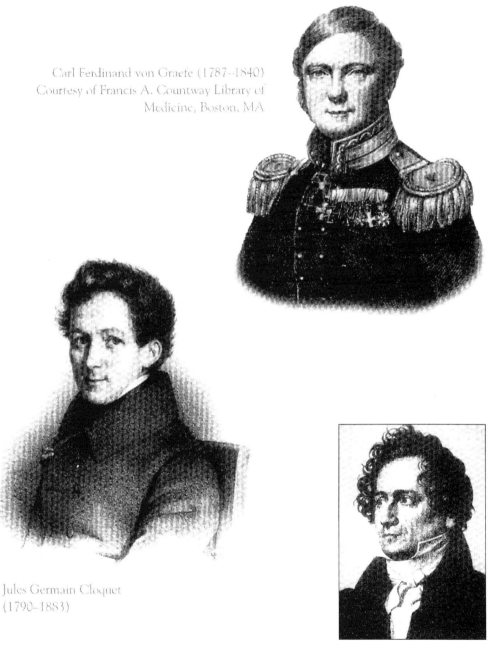

Carl Ferdinand von Graefe (1787–1840)
Courtesy of Francis A. Countway Library of
Medicine, Boston, MA

Jules Germain Cloquet
(1790–1883)

Johann Dieffenbach
(1792–1847)

1821   JAMES WILSON (1778–1845), a popular blind poet, published *Biography of the blind, or the lives such as have distinguished themselves as poets, philosophers, artists, etc.* Wilson was born in Richmond, Virginia, and at age four lost his parents and his eyesight to smallpox during a voyage to England.

1821   The New York Eye and Ear Infirmary was established by EDWARD DELAFIELD (1794–1875) and JOHN KEARNEY RODGERS (1793–1851), two young American physicians who had studied at Moorfields. Their infirmary was an immediate success and was the first institution in the United States to train ophthalmologists.

1821   LADY LOWTHER of York, England, whose son, SIR CHARLES, was blind, introduced the embossed texts of Valentin Haüy into England to enable her son to read.

1821   Chen Hou-His of China published *Yen K'e Liu Yao (The Six Essences of Ophthalmology)*. His book covered diseases and cures, including a description of clamping the lids with the aid of bamboo forceps for the treatment of trichiasis and entropion.

1821   BARTOLOMEO PANIZZA (1785–1867) contributed the first report of an enucleation for retinoblastoma.

1823–1847   JOHANN DIEFFENBACH (1792–1847) of Berlin, one of the founders of modern plastic surgery, performed extensive experiments to test Reisinger's idea of keratoplasty. None of his animal trials resulted in a perfect graft of the transplanted tissue, and Dieffenbach was not able to perfect the operation.

1823   JOHANN GOTTLIEB FABINI (1791–1847), ophthalmology professor at the University of Pest, published what was probably the final ophthalmology text in Latin, *Doctrina de morbis oculorum*. Fabini was director of Pest's institute for the indigent blind and contributed to the surgical treatment of strabismus.

1823   SIR CHARLES BELL, the leading British anatomist of his day, described in detail the motions of the human eye, the function of the ocular muscles, and the nerves of the orbit in his *On the motions of the eye*.

1823   GEORGE FRICK (1793–1870) of Baltimore published *A Treatise on the diseases of the eye*, based on the lectures of his teacher, Georg Beer of Vienna. This is the first American textbook of ophthalmology.

1823–1825   JAN EVANGELISTA PURKINJE, now at Breslau, published *Beobachtungen und Versuche zur Physiologie der Sinne*, which detailed that luminescence could be induced in eyes with reflected light from his spectacles. It seems likely he actually observed the fundus oculi decades before Helmholtz. He also noted the existence of the

Purkinje images and adopted an illuminated microscope to study the structure of the human iris. Purkinje's other contributions include the development of new visual field testing, as well as methods of preparing, fixing, and staining tissues.

1823   GEORGE JAMES GUTHRIE of London, an army surgeon in the Napoleonic Wars, published *Lectures on the operative surgery of the eye*, considered the first systematic English textbook on ophthalmic surgery. The book included a discussion on the diagnosis of eyelid tumors. Guthrie independently noted elevated intraocular pressure in glaucoma.

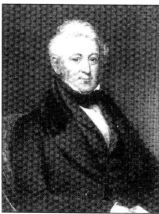

George James Guthrie (1785–1856)
Courtesy of Francis A. Countway Library of Medicine, Boston, MA

1824   FRIEDRICH HERMANN DE LEUW (1792–1861) of Gräfrath, Germany, published *Ueber die jetz herrschende contagiöse sogenannte egyptische Augenkrankheit* on trachoma.

1824   WILLIAM KITCHINER (1775?–1827) of London published his popular work *The economy of the eyes*. The book offered advice on the selection of eyeglasses, judging the quality of lenses, and described a 'pancratic eye tube' that Kitchiner invented for telescopes and microscopes.

1824   EDWARD REYNOLDS and JOHN JEFFERIES (1796–1876), both of Boston, founded the Massachusetts Charitable Eye and Ear Infirmary in that city.

1824   FRANZ REISINGER of Augsburg, the first to suggest the use of living tissue to take the place of opaque corneas (1818), experimented with the first keratoplasties on animal corneas. He excised the host cornea with a cataract knife and scissors and sutured in place a corneal graft. Although none of the grafts remained clear, healing occurred, and Reisinger concluded that a 'plastic process' had taken place.

1824   WILLIAM LAWRENCE (1783–1867), chief surgeon at St. Bartholomew's

Hospital in London, began giving lectures on eye diseases at Moorfields that helped ophthalmology to be viewed as a legitimate field of medicine. These lectures were published in *The Lancet*.

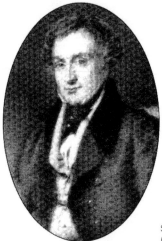

Sir William Lawrence
(1783–1867)

1824   WILLIAM EDMONDS HORNER (1793–1853) of Philadelphia, later professor of anatomy at the University of Pennsylvania, discovered the tensor tarsi (Horner's muscle) and described its function in compressing the puncta lacrimalia and lacrimal sac.

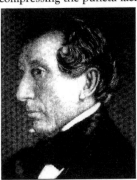

William Edmonds Horner
(1793–1853)

1825   GUISEPPE MARIA CANELLA (1788–1829), an ophthalmologist and surgeon in Trentino, Italy, established the *Giornale di chirurgia practica*. The journal covered the topics of general surgery and ophthalmic surgery.

1825   JEAN FRANÇOIS VLEMINCKX (1800–1876), a general practitioner in Brussels wrote *Essais sur l'Ophthalmie des Pays Bas* with CHARLES VAN MONS. They claimed the cause of military trachoma to be compression of the veins of the head and neck by soldiers' uniform collars and helmets. A number of physicians embraced this theory, and a controversy ensued between the 'compressionists' and the 'contagionists.'

1825   CARL HEINRICH WELLER of Dresden published *Icoues ophthalmologicae seu selecta circa morbos humani oculi*, an atlas containing case histories and illustrations of glaucoma, cataract, retinoblastoma, and vitreous floaters. Weller independently noted the association of elevated intraocular pressure with glaucoma.

c. 1826   JOSEPH JACKSON LISTER (1786–1869) modified the compound microscope to its modern form, which includes achromatic objectives.

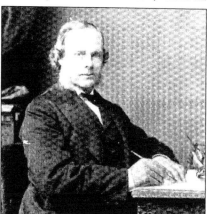

Joseph Jackson Lister (1786–1869)
Courtesy of Francis A. Countway Library of Medicine, Boston, MA

1826   WILLIAM CLEOBUREY (1793–1853), a surgeon to Oxford University and the city's leading ophthalmologist, published *A review of the different operations performed on the eyes of the restoration of lost and the improvement of imperfect vision*. Discussion covered several procedures for constructing an artificial pupil and several procedures for cataract operations, including extraction, discission, and depression.

1826   PHILIPP FRANZ VON WALTHER, professor of ophthalmology at Bonn, gave an early account of tarsorrhaphy. He subsequently was professor in Münich where he published *System der Chirurgie* (1833–1852), the fourth volume of which focused mainly on ophthalmic plastic surgery. This volume was reprinted as *Lehre von den Augenkrnakheiten* in 1849.

1826–1830   JUSTUS WILHELM MARTIN RADIUS (1797–1884), ophthalmology professor at the University of Leipzig, published his encyclopedic work *Scriptores ophthalmologici minores*. This is a compilation of the works of Baerens, Jaeger, von Walther, Martini, La Harpe, Schopenhauer, Jacobson and Richter, and others.

1826   JOHANNES MÜLLER (1801–1858) provided his explanation of color sensations produced by pressure on the retina in his *Zur vergleichenden*

Physiologie des Gesichtssinnes des Menschen. This work contained his 'law of specific nerve energies,' which states that humans do not perceive the process of the external world but only the effects they produce on their sensory systems. In the same year, Müller, in explaining the mechanics of eye movements, maintained that the globe moved only around a fixed point at the center of its posterior surface.

1826   JEAN DUBREUIL (1790–1852), a noted French cataract surgeon, published *The practice of perspective.*

1827   JOHN MCALLISTER was the first American optician to correct astigmatism by grinding plano-cylindrical lenses.

1827   ARTHUR JACOB, an ophthalmologist in Dublin, was the first to clinically identify basal cell carcinoma.

1827   JAMES GALL, a printer and philanthropist in Edinburgh improved the types Haüy invented for use in books for the blind by replacing all curves with straight lines. Using his new types, he issued parts of the Bible for publication. He later further modified the types, forming letters with dots to reduce the cost.

1827   EUGENE SCHNEIDER (1895–1874), a surgeon and professor of anatomy in Landshut, Germany, published *Das Ende der Nervenhaut im menschlichen Auge.* This provided an important early anatomical study of the ora serrata.

1827   SIR GEORGE BIDDELL AIRY (1801–1892), Lucasian Professor of Mathematics at Cambridge, ascertained the existence of astigmatism in his eye, which he continued to study over the course of almost 60 years. Airy is also responsible for introducing the term 'astigmatism' into the literature.

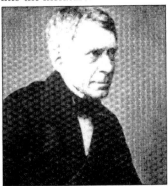

Sir George Biddell Airy
(1801–1892)

1827   PIERRE PREVOST of Geneva popularized use of the word 'Daltonism' to describe color blindness. This was subsequently largely replaced by the term color blindness, introduced by Sir David Brewster.

1827   THOMAS RICHARDSON COLLEDGE founded a 40-bed ophthalmic hospital in Macao, China, which handled 6000 cases during its operation until 1832.

1827   NATHANIEL MILLER of Massachusetts published the first report of cataract extraction in the United States (*A dissertation on the importance and manner of detecting deep seated matter*) in Boston. Miller was an active cataract surgeon, and he stated that in May and June of 1798 he operated on 21 eyes by extraction.

1828   JOHANN CHRISTIAN JÜNGKEN (1793–1875) appointed director of the Berlin Charity Hospital ophthalmology clinic. Jüngken, a renowned surgeon and teacher, was the first to perform ophthalmic surgery under general anesthesia.

1828   JOHN RICHARD FARRE (1774–1862), co-founder of the Royal London Ophthalmic Hospital (Moorfields), established the *Journal of Morbid Anatomy, Ophthalmic Medicine, and Pharmaceutical Analysis*. Farre amassed an enormous collection of pathological-anatomical specimens, many related to ophthalmology, and described interesting and unusual cases in his journal.

1828   BURKHARD EBLE (1799–1839), an Austrian military physician, published *Ueber den Bau und die Krankheiten der Bindehaut des Auges*. This is a detailed study of microscopic anatomy and pathology of the conjunctiva based on the author's research and observations in dealing with trachoma.

1828   DETMAR WILHELM SOEMMERRING of Frankfurt am Main published *Beobachtungen über die organischen Veränderungen im Auge nach Staaroperationen*. This is an investigation of structural changes in the eye following cataract surgery and is Soemmerring's most important ophthalmologic contribution. He reports on postmortem examinations of eight eyes that had been operated on previously for cataract. Ring-shaped masses of lens material (Soemmerring-ring cataracts) are described, which he regards as a regeneration of lens fibers produced by the capsule and its epithelium.

1828   WILHELM RAU (1804–1861), professor of ophthalmology and pediatrics at the University of Bern, published his work on staphyloma *Ueber die Erkenntniss, Entstehung und Heilung der Staphylome des menschlichen Auges*. Rau also published on iritis, *Die Krankheiten und Bildungsfehler der Regenbogenhaut* (1844–1845).

1828   AMMI PHILLIPS, an itinerant 'folk' artist in New York state, painted the first known American portrait of a surgeon performing eye surgery. The surgeon depicted was PETER BENNETT GUERNSEY

(1804–1873) of New York who is holding a corneal knife in preparation for cataract surgery.

1828   JOHANN MATTHIAS SCHOEN (1800–1870), a physician in Halle, Germany, published *Handbuch der pathologishen Anatomie des menschlichen Auges*. This thorough and systematic work discusses the pathologic anatomy of lesions involving the entire eyeball; pathologic changes in specific tissues; and finally, the 'formation of stones' and presence of worms in the eye.

1828   GOTTFRIED REINHOLD TREVIRANUS (1776–1839), a physician and microscopist in Bremen, published *Beiträge zur Anatomie und Physiologie der Sinneswerkzeuge des Menschen und der Thiere*. He formulated mathematical laws of diffraction and attempted to determine the mechanism responsible for our seeing things in their relative position. He also tried to define the functions of the cornea, lens, and retina. Treviranus published an additional work (1835–1837) on physiologic optics.

1828   ALBRECHT VON GRAEFE (1828–1870), the greatest eye surgeon of the nineteenth century, was born in Berlin, the son of the distinguished surgeon, Carl Ferdinand von Graefe.

1828   FRIEDRICH AUGUST VON AMMON (1799–1861) was appointed professor of pathology, clinical medicine, and surgery at Dresden's Medical-Surgical Academy and focused on ophthalmic plastic surgery. His contributions included descriptions of a cantholysis for entropion, full thickness triangle excision for ectropion, treatment of lacrimal system disease, surgical advancement for strabismus, correction of congenital ocular defects, and cure of symblepharon.

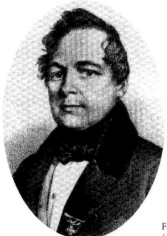

Friedrich August von Ammon
(1799–1861)

1829   SIR CHARLES BELL of Edinburgh demonstrated that the fifth cranial nerve is a sensory motor nerve.

1829   The United States' first institution for the blind was established and named the Perkins Institute in honor of the individual who had donated his mansion to the institution. SAMUEL G. HOWE was appointed its director in 1831, and he focused on advancing the education of the blind. Howe linked to teaching the blind the education of the deaf, as well. His methods were used for the education of Helen Keller and Laura Bridgeman.

1829   JOHANN KARL GEORGE FRICKE (1790–1841) published his pioneering monograph on reconstructive surgery of the eyelids, *Die Bildung neuer Augenlieder (Blepharoplastik) nach Zerstörungen*. Fricke includes a description of the use of pedicle flaps from the temple and cheek to achieve eyelid reconstruction.

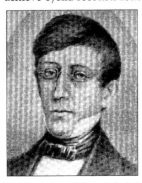

George Frick
(1793–1870)

1829   LOUIS SALOMON FALLOT (1783–1872), a Belgian ophthalmologist who served in the army under Napoleon, published an early work on Egyptian ophthalmia (trachoma), in which he theorized that the condition was contagious. Fallot was elected to serve as president of the First International Congress of Ophthalmology in Brussels in 1857.

1829   JOHANN FRIEDRICH DIEFFENBACH published *Chirurgische Erfahrungen besonders über die Widerherstallung Zerstörter Theile des menschlichen Körpers nach neuen Methoden*. His work describes many of his significant contributions to ophthalmic plastic surgery.

1830   SALOMON JAKOB SALOMON (1801–1862), in Schleswig, published a work on intraocular foreign bodies.

1830   JOHN FEARN (1768–1837), an English philosopher, published *A rationale of the laws of cerebral vision*. This deals with the physiology of vision in the context of consciousness, cognition, and sensory perception.

1830   ANTOM EDLER VON ROSAS (1791–1855), Chair of Ophthalmology in Vienna, published *Handbuch der theoretischen und practischen Augenheilkunde*. This 1500-page work was Rosas's major publication and in its time was the most comprehensive textbook of ophthalmology in the world. Rosas, a superb teacher of surgical ophthalmology, was also the inventor of several important instruments.

1830   JOHANN FRIEDERICH DANIEL LOBSTEIN (1777–1840) spent most of his life as a general practitioner and ophthalmologist in Strasbourg. His last years were spent in New York, where he published *A treatise upon the semiology of the eye*. This was actually a translation of a treatise by Löbenstein-Löel written in 1817 on the symptomatology of the eye.

1830   WILLIAM MACKENZIE, an influential Scottish ophthalmologist, published *A practical treatise on diseases of the eye*. This text was, with Lawrence's textbook, the leading English ophthalmic work of its time. In it MacKenzie differentiated for the first time glaucomatous amaurosis from cataract, noting that increased intraocular pressure is characteristic of glaucoma. Mackenzie also includes the first complete description of sympathetic ophthalmitis.

1830   WILLIAM LAWRENCE of London published *Treatise on venereal diseases of the eye* discussing the nature, symptoms, and treatment of venereal diseases affecting the eyes, including gonorrheal inflammation of the conjunctiva.

1830   The United States became the first country to formally count the cases of blindness in the course of its 1830 census. Since 1830, an enumeration of blind inhabitants has been made with each population census.

1830   JOSEPH FRANCIS MALGAIGNE (1806–1865), the French surgeon, published *Nouvelle théorie de la vision*. He bitterly opposed the separation of ophthalmology from general surgery. Malgaigne also advocated the couching of cataracts, claiming that only two out of 180 persons are innately ambidextrous and capable of doing extraction.

1830   FRIEDRICH SCHLEMM (1795–1858), professor of anatomy in Berlin, discovered the canal, which bears his name (canal of Schlemm), in the eye of a hanged criminal. He published an illustration of the canal in *Arteriarum capitis superficialium icon nova* but misidentified its exact location. In the same year he also discovered the corneal nerves.

1830   The Medical Faculty of Munich offered a prize for the best work on keratoplasty, and this served to stimulate much of the experimentation that followed during the next decade.

1830   VICTOR STOEBER (1803–1871) initiated the first university course in ophthalmology in France. This was in the University of Strasbourg where he served as professor of pathology.

1831   SIR DAVID BREWSTER of Edinburgh published *A treatise on optics*, which includes sections on catoptrics, physical optics, the application of optical principles, and optical instruments.

1831   HUMPHREY LLOYD (1800–1881), a Dublin physicist, published *A treatise on light and vision*. He discusses theories of simple light and compound light, dispersion of light by combining prisms or lenses, and theories of achromatism and color. Lloyd also includes laws of vision. His optical discoveries gave new support to the wave theory of light and expanded knowledge of the properties of reflection and refraction.

1831   ALEXANDER WATSON (1799–1879), an Edinburgh surgeon and ophthalmologist, founded the Royal Eye Infirmary in that city. His principal publications dealt with forensic medicine and anatomy of the eye.

1831   JOHANN MATTHIAS SCHOEN in Hamburg was the first to explain the pathology of arcus senilis, an abnormality that had been identified since ancient times.

1832   FRIEDRICH GUSTAV JAKOB HENLE (1809–1885) published *De membrana pupillari*, a handbook on the membrane of the pupil. Henle became the foremost German histologist of his time, making major discoveries in the histology of the cornea, lens, brain, and kidney.

1832   FRIEDRICH ARNOLD (1803–1890), an anatomy and physiology professor at Heidelberg, published *Anatomische und physiologische Untersuchunger über das Auge des Menschen*. This includes the location of the nerves of the iris, what he described as corneal lymphatic channels (actually the corneal nerves). Arnold's ganglion, Arnold's fold, and Arnold's membrane are named after him.

1832   SIR CHARLES WHEATSTONE, an English scientist, invented the stereoscope. This instrument provided popular amusement throughout the Victorian era.

1832   JOHANN NEPOMUK FISCHER (1777–1847) of Prague, considered the founder of modern ophthalmology in Bohemia, published *Klinischer Unterricht in der Augenheilkunde*. Fischer is the first, since the old Greek and Arab authors, to present a satisfactory description of trachoma in a textbook.

1832   JOHN MASON GIBSON, a Maryland surgeon, published the badly flawed second American work on ophthalmology (after Frick), *A condensation of matter upon the anatomy, surgical operations and treatment of disease of eye.* It was, however, the first American book on ophthalmology to include illustrations of eye disease.

1832   JULES SICHEL (1802–1868) founded the first eye clinic in Paris, a private institution on the rue Cloître St. Benoit that became a major center for research and education.

1832   JÖNS JACOB BERZELIUS (1779–1848), Swedish physician and chemist, used chemical analysis to study the composition of the aqueous humor.

1833   JOSEPH PLATEAU (1801–1883), a physiologist at Ghent, introduced cinematography and studied color vision, stroboscopy, afterimages, and contrast phenomena.

1833   DETMAR WILHELM SOEMMERRING published the first account of a living cysticercus in a human eye.

1833   BURKHARD WILHELM SEILER (1779–1843), director of the Medical-Surgical Academy of Dresden, published *Beobachtungen urspruenglicher Bildungsfehler und gaezlichen Mangels der Augen*. This was the earliest monograph on congenital ocular anomalies, and Seiler provided interpretations for these according to the general laws of organogenesis as it was then understood.

1833   ALEXANDER FRIEDRICH HUECK (1802–1842), an anatomist and physiologist at Dorpat, published *Das Sehen*, an important work on the physiology of the eye.

1833   BENEDICT STILLING (1810–1879) of Kassel, Germany, in his *Die kunstliche Pupillen bildung in der Sclerotica*, described his successful transplantation in rabbits of corneal tissue into an opening in the sclera. The transplanted cornea healed in place and remained transparent. He also experimented with sectioning the eye by freezing it in a brine solution.

1833   WILHELM TOHMÉ (b.1809) of Bonn wrote *De Corneae Transplantation*. He attempted eight experimental keratoplasties using a spear-shaped knife of his own design and a single incision.

1833   SIR CHARLES BELL of Edinburgh described the motor nerve of the face (portio dura of the seventh nerve), lesions of which cause facial paralysis (Bell's palsy). Discussion of this is contained in his *The nervous system of the human body*.

1833   SIR WILLIAM LAWRENCE published *Treatise on the diseases of the eye*. This comprehensive work represented a milestone in the teaching of ophthalmic surgery.

1833–1836   CHRISTIAN GOTTFRIED EHRENBERG (1795–1875) of Berlin published the results of the first detailed microscopic study of the retina. Using primitive fixation and lacking embedding and staining techniques, he concluded that the retina was similar to the brain in being composed of fine fibers continuous with those of the optic nerve and containing a whitish medullary layer.

1833   SIR JOHN HARRISON CURTIS (b. 1778), a London ophthalmologist and otologist, published *A treatise on the physiology and diseases of the eye, containing a new mode of curing cataract.* One of the best descriptions of ocular physiology and comparative ophthalmic anatomy since Aristotle and As-Sadili. Curtis discusses experiments on vision, preservation of sight, and the need for spectacles to correct errors in vision.

1834   JOHN WALKER (1803?–1847), a surgeon at the Manchester Eye Infirmary in England, published *The principles of ophthalmic surgery.* This gave clear descriptions of the principal eye diseases and the accepted mode of treatment at the time.

1834   MARIA HACK (1777–1844) of Southampton, England published her *Lectures at home. Discovery and manufacture of glass: lenses and mirrors: the structure of the eye.* Hack was a writer of popular science and history books for children.

1834   VICTOR STOEBER of Strasbourg published *Manuel pratique d'ophthalmologie ou traité des maladies des yeux.* This was the best French text of its time.

1834   JOHN DALRYMPLE (1803–1852), an assistant surgeon to the Royal London Ophthalmic Hospital (Moorfields), published *The anatomy of the human eye.* This was the first English work on ocular anatomy and was modeled after Johann Zinn's text of 1755. His work provided invaluable information in orbital anatomy and basic surgical technique. Dalrymple's sign in exopthalmic goiter is named for him.

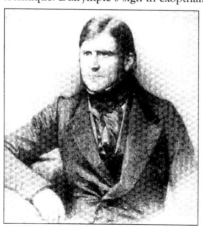

John Dalrymple
(1803–1852)

1834	Two Spanish surgeons, DIEGO DE ARGUMOSA Y OBREGON (1792–1865) and JOAQUIN HYSERN Y MOLLARIS (1804–1883), both published works on eyelid reconstruction successfully using Dieffenbach's technique.
1834	JULES SICHEL, a major contributor to modern French ophthalmic plastic surgery, promoted a method of eyelid reconstruction using a flap from the arm.
1834	JAMES GALL published A historical sketch of the origin and progress of literature for the blind containing practical recommendations for educating the blind.
1835	PETER PARKER (1804–1889), a graduate of Yale University in medicine and theology, a Protestant medical missionary and late diplomat, opened and directed a hospital in Canton, China, specializing in the treatment of eye diseases, particularly cataract.
1835	GABRIEL GUSTAV VALENTIN (1810–1883), professor of physiology and comparative anatomy professor at Bern, published Lehrbuch der Physiologie des Menschen which includes many of his observations on the anatomy and physiology of the eye.
1835	RICHARD MIDDLEMORE (1840–1896), surgeon at Birmingham Eye Hospital, published A treatise on the diseases of the eye and its appendages. Middlemore, renowned for his benefactions, also established an ophthalmology prize (1877) awarded by the British Medical Association, established and supported the Birmingham Asylum for the Blind, and endowed a course of lectures at Birmingham and Midland Eye Hospital (1888).
1835	CHARLES JOSEPH FRÉDÉRIC CARRON DU VILLARDS published Recherches pratiques sur les causes cui font échouer l'opération de la cataracte, which analyzes the cataract operation, its successes, and the accidents involved. Du Villards lived for periods in North Africa, Mexico, and Central and South America and wrote extensively on tropical eye diseases.
1835	GEORG HEERMANN (1807–1844) at Heidelberg published Über die Bildung der Gesichtsvorstelungen aus den Gesichtsempfindungen on visual perception.
1836	ALFRED WILHELM VOLKMANN (1800–1877) suggested that the eye moved around a point at its center, contradicting Johannes Müller's earlier (1826) concept that the globe only moved around a fixed point at the center of its posterior surface.
1836	New York ophthalmologist WILLIAM CLAY WALLACE, published The structure of the eye with reference to natural theology, an important

treatise on the comparative anatomy of the eye and the physiology of vision. Wallace was opposed to the wearing of glasses.

1836   BERNHARD RUDOLPH KONRAD LANGENBECK (1810–1887) published *De retina: observationes anatomico-pathologicae*. He presents microscopic proof that neoplasms of the retina consist essentially of a hyperplasia of the normal retinal cells.

1837   SQUIRE LITTELL (1803–1886) published *Manual on diseases of the eye*, based on his experience at the Wills Hospital and in private practice. The *Manual* was the first American book to be based exclusively on the author's clinical experiences.

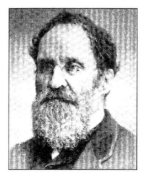

Squire Littell
(1803–1886)

1837   LUDWIG FRIEDRICH SEEBECK (1805–1849), a physicist in Berlin, carried out studies of color blindness that led him to classify color blindness into two groups: one who had 'full length spectra vision' and one who had 'shortened spectra vision.'

1837   S. L. L. BIGGER, an Irishman, published a report describing his successful attempt at keratoplasty. It detailed replacing the scarred corneas of a pet gazelle that he performed while held captive by Bedouins in the Sahara Desert. The donor cornea was taken from another animal, and the superior portion of the cornea remained clear.

1837   WILLIAM EDMONDS HORNER, professor of anatomy at the University

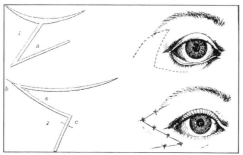

Z-plasty
(Horner)

of Pennsylvania, advanced basic plastic surgery with the Z-plasty or 'switch flap' technique.

1837   ALESSANDRO RIBERI (1794–1861), the first professor of ophthalmology at Turin, described a new procedure for the correction of ectropion of the lower lid. Two skin incisions are made from the external and also from the nasal canthus along the palpebral margin. They meet below at an obtuse angle. The skin flap is dissected and the lid margin lifted. The triangular flap is implanted in the upper half of the defect.

1837–1840   JOHANNES MÜLLER, the founder of modern experimental physiology, now in Berlin, published *Handbuch der Physiologie des Menschen*. This contained a critical examination of existing knowledge and important new findings on visual physiology.

1838   The first of the four parts of FRIEDRICH AUGUST VON AMMON'S atlas *Klinische Darstellungen der Krankheiten des menschlichen Auges* (1838–1847) is issued. This magnificent work provides clinical descriptions and illustrations of the diseases and congenital anomalies of the human eye, lids, and lacrimal system.

1838   CHARLES JOSEPH FRÉDÉRIC CARRON DU VILLARDS of Paris published *Guide pratique pour l'étude et le traitement des maladies des yeux*. This is one of the best books of the period on the diagnosis and treatment of diseases of the eye. Carron du Villards describes his galvano-puncture method for removal of displaced, particularly inverted, cilia.

1838   CASIMIR SPERINO (1812–1894) established the first outpatient eye clinic in Turin, which in 1853 became an eye hospital. Sperino also published a notable paper advocating intracapsular cataract extraction and defended this with statistical studies (1858).

1838   FLORENT CUNIER (1812–1853), one of the founders of Belgian ophthalmology and an innovative ophthalmic surgeon, initiated the Belgian journal *Annales d'Oculistique*.

1838   GEORGE COX in England published *Spectacle Secrets*, which described a system for determining the needed spectacle lens strength and contributed to our development of the modern trial case. Cox's trial case consisted of eight pairs of spectacles of known power to be used in carrying out a refractive examination.

1838   GEORG HEERMANN of Heidelberg published his study on the dreams of blind persons.

1838   EDUARD ZEIS (1807–1868), a pioneer plastic surgeon and ophthalmologist in Dresden, published *Handbuch der Plastichen Chirurgie*. This introduced the term 'plastic surgery' and was the first complete book on this subject. Zeis was noted for his skill in performing blepharoplasty and strabismus operations.

1838   GEORGE FRIEDRICH LOUIS STROMEYER (1804–1876), a military surgeon in Germany, proposed myotomy of the internal rectus muscle as a treatment for strabismus, reporting that he had experimented with the procedure on cadavers.

1838   LOUIS JOSEPH SANSON, Sr. (1790–1843) published *Leçons des maladies des yeux*. He employed Purkinje's findings of three lens images (1823) diagnostically, and as a result these became known as the Purkinje–Sanson images.

1839   MICHEL EUGÈNE CHEVREUL (1786–1889), a special professor of chemistry at the Gobelins in France, published *De la loi du contraste simultané des couleurs, et de l'assortiment des objets colorés*. He discusses in detail the topics of color contrast and human conception of color. This was one of the most influential treatises on color of the nineteenth century.

1839   FRANCESCO ROGNETTA (1800–1857), trained in Naples and practicing in Paris, published *Cours d'ophthalmologie*. He recommends belladonna, colomel, and strychnine for amaurosis and optic nerve disease. Rognetta established a course in ophthalmology.

1839   FRÉDÉRIC JOSEPH HAIRION (1809–1887), an ophthalmology professor at Leuven, published *Considérations pratiques et recherches expérimentales sur le traitement de l'ophthalmie*. Hairion espoused the popular view that trachoma and other infectious diseases were spread through both miasmata and contagion. He discusses extensively the ophthalmic use of tannin. In the same year he founded an institute for soldiers with eye diseases (Institute ophthalmique militaire).

1839   JOHANN FRIEDRICH DIEFFENBACH of Berlin was the first to perform an ocular muscle-sectioning procedure for the correction of strabismus on a living subject.

1839   THEODOR SCHWANN (1810–1882), working in the department of JOHANNES MÜLLER, reported that Schleiden's plant cell theory was also true for animals.

1840–1849   FLORENT CUNIER established the first ophthalmic clinic in Brussels. Cunier began testing patients' eyesight through the use of a set of test lenses in frames.

1840   THÉOPHILE DROUOT (1830–1886), a well-known Parisian ophthalmologist, published *Nouveau traité des cataractes*. It describes his treatment of cataract consisting of the use of quinine, potassium iodide, belladonna, or aconite, depending on the symptoms present in each eye.

1840   FREDERICK TYRRELL (1793–1843), a highly skilled ophthalmic surgeon at London Eye Infirmary and St. Thomas' Hospital, published *A practical work on the diseases of the eye, and their treatment, medically, topically, and by operation*. This book was notable for its 143 detailed case histories.

1840   GUSTAV THEODOR FECHNER (1801–1887), the founder of psychophysics in Germany, emphasized the relationship between contrast and the effects of juxtapositioning complementary colors. Fechner also investigated the causes and nature of afterimages.

1840   FRANZ XAVER MÜHLBAUER of Munich published *Über Transplantation der Cornea*. He noted that he tried experimental penetrating grafts without success and consequently turned his attention to Walther's proposal to transplant the anterior corneal layers only. Mühlbauer cut triangular partial thickness grafts that were held in place by a suture and the pressure of the eyelids.

1840   ADOLPHE HANNOVER (1814–1894) of Copenhagen discovered the ganglion cells of the retina.

1841   CARL FRIEDRICH GAUSS (1777–1855), mathematician and director of Göttingen's observatory, published *Dioptrische Untersuchungen*. Gauss analyzes the path of light through a system of lenses. His results show that any system is equivalent to a properly chosen single lens.

1841   SALVATORE FURNARI (1808–1866), professor of ophthalmology at the University of Palermo, published *Traité pratique des maladies des yeux*. Funari discusses occupational diseases and hygiene as they relate to the eye.

1841   BADEN POWELL (1796–1860), physicist and professor of geometry at Oxford, published *A general and elementary view of the undulatory theory*. Powell presents his studies on light dispersion and radiant heat, which support the wave theory of light.

1841   JOHN HOMER DIX (1813–1884) of Boston, one of the founders of the American Ophthalmological Society, published *Treatise on strabismus, or squinting, and the new mode of treatment*. Dix was the first American to perform Dieffenbach's operation for strabismus.

1841   JOSEPH FRIEDRICH PIRINGER (1800–1879), professor of ophthalmology in Graz, published *Die Blennorrhoe am Menschenauge*. Piringer treated Pannus trachomatosus with the discharge of blennorrhea of the newborn.

1841   CHARLES PHILLIPS (1811–1870) of Liege, Belgium published *Du bégaiement et du strabisme, nouvelles recherches* and *De la tenotomie sous-cutanée*. Phillips, after relocating to St. Petersburg, operated on 300

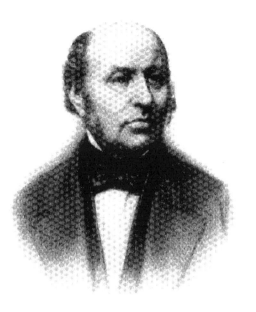

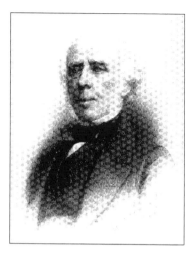

Sir William Mackenzie (1791–1868)
Courtesy of Francis A. Countway Library of
Medicine, Boston, MA

Jules Sichel
(1802–1868)

Carl Friedrich Gauss
(1777–1855)

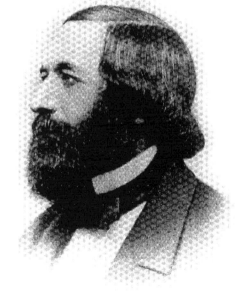

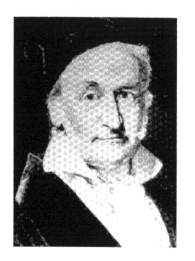

John Dix
(1813–1884)

patients for strabismus, and he describes the several methods he employed.

1841   ALFRED CHARLES POST (1806–1886), surgeon at the College of Physicians and Surgeons in New York City, published *Observations on the cure of strabismus*. He was one of the first American to operate for strabismus. Post discusses his methods and results and includes several colored plates. He also performed early blepharoplasty surgery (1842).

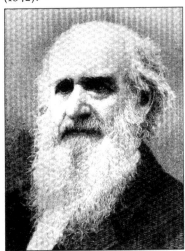

Alfred Charles Post
(1806–1886)

1841   T. KÖNIGSHOFER published *De transplantatione corneae* that detailed his animal experiments using the lamellar graft technique. He developed a double-edged knife and reported that ten of fourteen transplants healed with transparent lamellae. Königshofer also attempted transplantation of cadaveric human cornea to animal eyes.

1841   JACOBUS LUDOVICUS CONRADUS SCHOEDER VAN DER KOLK (1797–1862) of Utrecht contributed his *Reserches anatomico-pathologic sur l'inflammation de queques parties profondes l'oeil*. In it he suggests inflammation of the choroids as a cause of glaucoma. The meticulous gross pathologic anatomical studies were important in development of ocular pathology.

1841   AMÉDÉE BONNET (1802–1858) of Lyons, France and JOSEPH MICHAEL O'FERRALL (1790–1877) in Ireland independently published reports on enucleation that rediscovered and further describe Tenon's capsule. Bonnet's work in particular set the stage for modern enucleation.

1841   WILLIAM MACKENZIE of Glasgow published *The physiology of vision*, which gave an outline of the laws of vision, with an account of the iris, retina, and optic nerve. In the same year, he also contributed his *The cure of strabismus by surgical operation.*

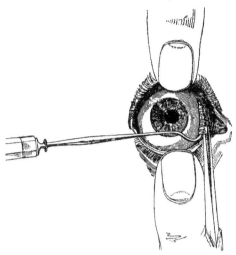

Illustration from *The cure of strabismus by surgical operation* (1841) by William Mackenzie

1841   GIOVANNI BATTISTA QUADRI delivered a lecture to the Académie Royale de Médicin in Paris on a new method of couching by depression he developed, following the principles described by Celsus, Albucasis, Avicenna, and Scarpa.

1842–1844   LUCIEN A.-H. BOYER (1808–1890), a Parisian physician and surgeon, published *Recherches sur l'opération de strabisme*. His work discusses the surgical treatment of strabismus and provides 100 case histories.

1842   FRIEDRICH AUGUST VON AMMON of Dresden published *Die plastiche Chirurgie*. Ammon described procedures for blepharoplasty and canthoplasty. The latter operation was modified by DAVID HAYES AGNEW at the University of Pennsylvania and became known as the Ammon–Agnew cantholysis.

1842   JOHANN FRIEDRICH DIEFFENBACH of Berlin published *Über das Schielen und die Heilung desselben durch die Operation*, which gave a full account of the author's method for correcting strabismus by severing the tendons of the eye muscles. He discussed the results of 1200 subsequent procedures. Although his muscle-cutting procedure met with initial enthusiasm, it was later abandoned owing to frequently disastrous final results.

1842   JAMES BOLTON (1812–1869) of Richmond, Virginia published *A treatise on strabismus, with a description of new instruments*. One of the early American texts on strabismus surgery, it presents Bolton's methods of operation with a description of the relevant anatomy and speculations on the causes of strabismus.

1842	SAMUEL MORITZ PAPPENHEIM (1811–1882) of Germany published the first book on the histology of the eye *Die specielle Gewebelehre des Auges mit Rücksicht auf Entwicklungsgeschichte und Augenpraxis*. This included a complete description of the corneal nerves first noted by Schlemm in 1830.
1842	ALFRED ARMAND LOUIS MARIE VELPEAU (1795–1867) of Paris published *Du strabisme*.
1842	JULES SICHEL of Paris published *Mémoire sur le glaucome*, the first monograph to focus on glaucoma. He theorized that glaucoma was a degeneration of the choroids due to its acute or chronic inflammation and that degeneration of the retina always accompanies this inflammation. He further stated that the treatment of glaucoma was that of choroiditis, and there was no verified case of a cured glaucoma.
1842	VICTOR STOEBER of Strasbough performed an enucleation in Strasbourg. Stoeber's method was subsequently refined and popularized by George Critchett at Moorfields Hospital and by William White Cooper at St. Mary's Hospital in London.
1843	KARL HIMLY, professor of medicine in Göttingen, claimed to have suggested the technique of keratoplasty to FRANZ REISINGER in 1824. Reisinger, nevertheless, is usually credited for suggesting replacing scarred corneas with living tissue.
1843	GEORGE FRONMÜLLER (1809–1889) invented a 'trial case' of 60 different trial lenses that fit into a special frame. This allowed the physician to select the correct glasses even if the patient's eyes had different refractions.
1843	HEINRICH KÜCHLER of Därmstadt Germany, developed a method for testing vision using a standard reading chart consisting of letters that diminished in size.
1843	JEAN JULIEN VAN ROOSBROECK (1810–1869) of Ghent published a 159-page monograph on ophthalmia neonatorum. In the same year, he published a paper attributing myopia to elongation of the eye.
1844	RICHARD SHARP KISSAM (1808–1861) of New York published an account in the *New York Journal of Medicine and the Collateral Sciences* of his 1838 operation in which, for the first time, an animal cornea was grafted to a human eye. The patient, James Dunn, had an immediate improvement in his vision, but two weeks later the cornea became opaque.
1844	FRANÇOIS LOUIS TAVIGNOT (b. 1818) of Paris is credited with coining

the term 'cyclitis' in reference to inflammation of the ciliary body.

1844   ADOLPHE HANNOVER introduced chromic acid fixation of tissues for histopathologic study. This solution again found use as a fixative with the advent of electron microscopy.

1844   JULES SICHEL of Paris gave the first accurate description of the herniated orbital fat associated with blepharochalasis.

1844   HORACE WELLS (1815–1848) introduced the use of nitrous oxide for anesthesia in dentistry but abandoned the practice after a fatal complication.

1844   JOHANN FRIEDRICH DIEFFENBACH of Berlin received the Paris Academy of Sciences' Monthyon Prize for being the first to successfully perform a tenotomy for strabismus on a living patient.

1844   CHARLES DEVAL (1806–1862), who practiced ophthalmology in Paris, published *Chirurgie oculaire*. This was only the second work in French devoted exclusively to eye surgery.

1844   GEORG EMANUEL JÄSCHE (1815–1876) of Dorpat, Estonia popularized a 3-stage operation for the treatment of trichiasis and distichiasis: (1) the ciliary margin is severed from the lid in its entire length excepting 2 bridges; (2) a crescent-shaped piece of skin is excised from the lid; (3) the severed lid margin is reattatched. This operation is essentially the same as that described by the ancient Greek surgeons Paulus of Aegina and Aëtius.

1845   FILIPPO PACINI (1812–1883) of Pisa published *Nuove ricerche microscopiche sulla tessitura intima della retina nell'uomo*. This gave the first complete and correct description of the layers of the retina.

1845   WILLIAM MOON (1818–1894) of England, himself blind, invented embossed Roman letters to enable blind persons to read.

1845   EDUARD ZEIS professor of surgery at Marburg published *Abhandlungen aus dem Gebiete der Chirurgie*. He discusses improved techniques for blepharoplasty and strabismus surgery. The 'glands of Zeis' are a reminder of his meticulous studies of the anatomy of the eyelid.

1845   FRANK HASTINGS HAMILTON (1813–1886), a surgeon and anatomist at the University of Buffalo, published *Monograph on strabismus, with cases*.

1845   ADOLF KUSSMAUL (1822–1902), while a student at Heidelberg, published *Die Farbenerscheinung im Grunde des menschlichen Auges* in which he demonstrated that the retina is transparent and is located 'at the focus of the refractive system of the eye.' This work presented groundbreaking studies on the luminosity of the pupil, through which Kussmaul came close to inventing the ophthalmoscope.

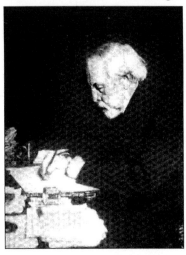

Adolf Kussmaul
(1822–1902)

1845   PLINY EARLY of Philadelphia reported the first cases of color blindness in America by detailing five generations of his own family with this disorder.

1845   JULES RENÉ GUÉRIN (1801–1886), an ophthalmologist and orthopedist in Paris, performed a successful subconjunctival myotomy surgery in the surgical treatment of strabismus. This was a major advance in the treatment of strabismus because the dangers of cellulitis and overcorrection were lessened.

1845   WILLIAM MACKENZIE published his study *Vision of objects on and in the eye*, a pioneer work in the field of catoptrics.

1845   JOHANN BENEDIKT LISTING (1808–1882), mathematician and physicist at the University of Göttingen, published *Beitrag zur physiologischen*

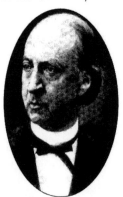

Johann Benedikt Listing
(1808–1882)

Optik. This discusses the anatomy and physiology of the eye, vision, and the properties of light. He originated the terms 'entoptic vision' and 'scintillating scotoma.' The same year, Listing gave an early explanation of hypermetropia 'as the condition in which the posterior focal point of the eye falls behind the retina.'

1845 CHRISTIAN GEORG THEODOR RUETE (1810–1867), while professor of medicine at Göttingen, published *Lehrbuch der Ophthalmologie*, containing a description of hypermetropia, which helped pave the way for Donder's discoveries.

1845 FRANÇOIS LOUIS TAVIGNOT of Paris published *Étude clinique sur les maladies de la cornée*, which classified and recommended therapies for the various types of acute and chronic keratitis.

1845–1848 JOHANN FRIEDRICH DIEFFENBACH of Berlin, the inventor of the strabismus operation in 1839, published *Die Operative Chirurgie*. This contains a detailed exposition of his methods of performing plastic surgery of the eye and elsewhere.

1846 CARL FERDINAND VON ARLT (1812–1887), an instructor at the University of Prague, published *Die Pflege der Augen im gesunden und kranken Zustande, nebst einen Anhange über Augengläser* intended for the lay public. He provides in this work hygienic and other protective considerations for eye care to be observed for the infant, the child, and the adult.

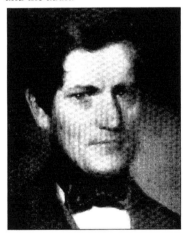

Carl Ferdinand von Arlt
(1812–1887)

1846 WILLIAM CUMMING (1817–1856), unaware of Purkinje's work in this field, published his findings that a reflex could be obtained from the fundus of the eye under certain conditions of illumination. Cummings also studied the change of the luminosity of the eye in various abnormal states. This was a significant preliminary study to the invention of the ophthalmoscope. He published his findings in an article entitled 'On a luminous appearance of the human eye and its application to the detection of disease of the retina and posterior part of the eye.'

1846 CRAWFORD W. LONG (1815–1578), of the University of Pennsylvania School of Medicine, began using ether anesthesia but did not publish his discovery until 1849.

1846 On October 16, JOHN COLLINS WARREN (1778–1856) of Harvard used ether anesthesia during the removal of a congenital vascular tumor of the neck. This was done at the urging of William Thomas Green Morton (1819–1868), a dental partner of Horace Wells who used nitrous oxide in dentistry. The eminent surgeon HENRY J. BIGELOW (1787–1879) published a report of the successful anesthesia operation performed by Warren. Because of the associated nausea and vomiting, however, ether found limited use in intraocular surgery, but it was widely employed for surgery of the orbit and adnexa.

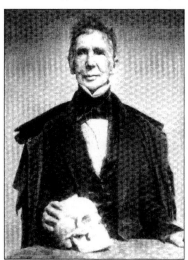

John Collins Warren
(1778–1856)

1847 WILLIAM MOON of England published his first book in Moon type. This used a system of embossed characters whose forms were simpler than those then in use. Moon raised funds for the printing and lending of embossed-type books, periodicals, maps, mathematical figures, and music and established schools and home teaching societies for the blind.

1847 ALFRED SMEE (1818–1877) of London, electrophysiologist and ophthalmologist, published *Vision in health and disease*. Smee founded an ophthalmic surgery clinic in London and was surgeon at the Central London Ophthalmic Institution.

1847 PIERRE ALEXANDRE CHARLES MAGNE (1818–1887) of Paris published *Hygiene de la vue*. He gives instructions on the care and hygiene of the eyes and the preservation of vision.

1847 FRANS CORNELIS DONDERS (1818–1889) of the University of Utrecht examined eye movements through the study of afterimages. He concluded: 'While no rolling component entered into purely horizontal and vertical movements, a torsion of after-image was observed in all oblique movements.' Donders also described the use of prismatic glasses in the treatment of strabismus.

1847 SIR JAMES YOUNG SIMPSON (1811–1870) introduced the use of chloroform anesthesia for obstetrics. JULIUS JACOBSON (1828–1889) in Königsberg was among the first to use chloroform in ophthalmic operations, and chloroform soon became the preferred general anesthetic for intraocular surgery.

1847 W. A. BALDWIN of the United States reported the experimental production of amblyopia with quinine.

1847 JOSEPH GERLACH (1820–1896) of Mainz noted that the nuclei distinctly take up alkaline carmine. This was an important early observation regarding tissue staining and was utilized in eye pathology.

1847 SIR WILLIAM BOWMAN (1816–1892), the renowned London ophthalmic anatomist, histologist, and surgeon, delivered a landmark series of lectures at Moorfields on the anatomy and histology of the eye. The lectures were collected and published the following year as *Lectures on the parts concerned in the operations on the globe and on the structure of the retina, delivered at the Royal London Ophthalmic Hospital, Moorfields: June 1847*. Among Bowman's discoveries are the anterior elastic lamina of the cornea (Bowman's membrane) and the structure of the ciliary muscles.

1847 WILLIAM WHITE COOPER (1816–1886), of North London Ophthalmic Institution and St. Mary's Hospital, Paddington, published *Practical remarks on near sight, aged sight, and impaired vision*. White discusses ocular structure, principles of light, reflection and refraction, treatment of myopia and presbyopia, and the consequences of artificial light on the eye.

1847 ERNST WILHELM VON BRÜCKE (1819–1892), professor of physiology at the University of Vienna, described his discovery of the phenomenon of luminosity of the eye in man in an article entitled 'Über das Leuchten der menschlichen Augen.' Helmholtz later remarked that Brücke 'was but a hair's breadth away from the invention of the ophthalmoscope.'

In the same year, Brücke published *Anatomische Beschreibung des menschlichen Augapfels*, an important study of ocular anatomy.

1847   ROBERT HAMILTON (d. 1868) of London, in a report entitled 'A case of imperfect vision from irregular refraction', confirmed Hirschel's and Brewster's claim that an asymmetrical cornea was the cause of astigmatism.

1847   CHARLES BABBAGE (1792–1871), a Cambridge mathematics professor, developed an instrument for examining the eye's interior, antedating Helmholtz's invention of the ophthalmoscope by three years. Babbage is best remembered for designing a machine that was the predecessor to the modern computer.

1847   THOMAS WHARTON JONES, professor of ophthalmology at University College Hospital, London, published *The principles and practice of ophthalmic medicine and surgery*. It was the last English textbook published before the introduction of the ophthalmoscope.

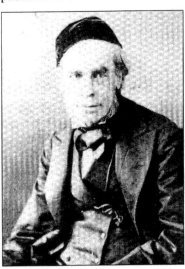

Thomas Wharton Jones (1808–1891)
Courtesy of Francis A. Countway Library of Medicine, Boston, MA

1847   Geneva Medical School in New York admitted ELIZABETH BLACKWELL in what was intended as a joke. This pioneer woman physician graduated in 1849 and continued her education in Europe. Blackwell found her way into ophthalmic history after fluid from an infant with gonorrheal ophthalmia squirted into her left eye. The eye eventually became blind and painful and was enucleated in 1850 by Louis Auguste Desmarres.

1847   LOUIS AUGUSTE DESMARRES (1810–1882) of France published *Traité théorique et pratique des maladies des yeux*. It includes the first systematic classification of orbital fractures, as well as discussions of diseases of the eyelids, the lacrimal glands, and the globe.

1847   FRANÇOIS LOUIS TAVIGNOT of Paris published *Traité clinicque des maladies des yeux*, which was notable for its thorough and precise description of cataract surgery and the formation of a new pupil.

1848   PHILIPP FRANZ VON WALTHER in Munich suggested the technique of a partial penetrating graft whereby only the anterior corneal layers were removed, with the deeper layers and Descemet's membrane left intact.

1848   SIR HENRY LAYARD (1817–1894) discovered the earliest known lens to date among the ruins of Nineveh. It is a plano-convex lens of rock crystal that is believed to date from the seventh century BC.

1848   SIR WILLIAM BOWMAN in London reported that the vitreous is made up of fibrils and granules clustered in bundles. His observation was subsequently confirmed by others, including Rudolph Virchow.

1848   JOHANN FRIEDRICH DIEFFENBACH in Berlin reported the successful treatment of involutional ectropion by means of lower lid reconstruction and tightening.

1849–1850   MAXIMILIAN ADOLPH LANGENBECK (1818–1877) of Göttingen published *Klinische Beiträge aus dem Gebiete der Chirurgie und Ophthalmologie*. The six sections on ophthalmology covered cataract extraction, the musculus compressor lentis, and ophthalmia. Lagenbeck reinvented the fixation forceps and brought this instrument into common use.

1849   CHARLES NICOLAS ALEXANDER HALDAT DU LYS (1770–1852) of Nancy, France published *Optique oculaire, suivie d'un essai sur l'achromatisme*, a significant work on the physiology of vision.

1849   SIR WILLIAM BOWMAN published a revised and expanded version of his *Lectures*. Among his new contributions are many surgical procedures, such as those for ptosis, lacrimal disorders, and formation of an artificial pupil. His inventions include lacrimal probes and suction-syringes for soft-cataract operations.

1849   GEORGE GABRIEL STOKES (1819–1903), a mathematician and physicist at Cambridge, invented the 'Stokes lens' to measure the degree of astigmatism. This device was a variable cylinder composed of plus and minus plano-cylinders of the same power and so constructed that they rotated in equal and opposite directions. It worked on the principle later utilized in cross-cylinder testing for astigmatism.

1849   EMIL DU BOIS-REYMOND (1818–1896), professor of physiology in Berlin, discovered that there was a 'current of rest' (resting potential) in the retina, similar to what he previously described in muscle and nerve. Du Bois-Reymond is considered a founder of modern electrophysiology.

1850 PIERRE ARMAND DUFAU (1795–1877), a French sociologist and advocate for the blind who served as instructor (1815) and later director (1840) of the Institution des Jeunes Aveugles, published *Des aveugles*. This covered the education of the blind using Braille's system of writing and musical notation and Haüy's cursive, which are illustrated and discussed.

1850 ALFRED VELPEAU, chief of the surgery clinic at the Charité in Paris, published *Manuel practique des maladies des yeux, d'apres les leçons cliniques d'Alfred Velpeau, par Gustave Jeanselme*. This was considered one of the most authoritative French works of the nineteenth century. Velpeau, a general surgeon, argued strongly against ophthalmology becoming a specialty.

1850 JOSEF VON HASNER (1819–1892) in Prague studied the anatomy, physiology, and pathology of the lacrimal system. He published his findings in *Berträge zur Physiologie und Pathologie des Thränenableitungsapparates*.

1850 The Women's Medical College of Pennsylvania was established by JOSEPH LONGSHORE. This marked the beginning of medical reform to include women and offered a venue for their training in medicine and its subspecialities, including diseases of the eye.

1850 AUGUST NÉLATON, professor of surgery at the University of Paris, published his famous treatise on cataract surgery, *Parallèle des divers modes opératoires employés dans le traitment de la cataracte*.

1851–1857 HEINRICH MÜLLER (1820–1864), professor of anatomy at Würzburg, began his pioneering studies on the histologic pathology of the eye. Over the next five years, he contributed many observations regarding papilledema, optic atrophy, glaucomatous cupping, drusen of the retina, drusen of the optic nerve, the nature of capsular cataracts,

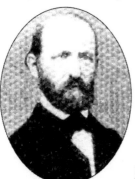

Heinrich Müller (1820–1864)
Courtesy of Francis A. Countway Library of Medicine, Boston, MA

histopathology of retinitis pigmentosa, and the nature of metastatic ophthalmia. He was of particular importance in correlating ophthalmoscopic observations with pathologic changes. Müller's cells, Müller's fibers, Müller's ciliary muscle, and Müller's muscle of the orbit are named for him.

1851 HERMANN VON HELMHOLTZ (1821–1894), physicist and physiologist, while an instructor of physiology at Königsberg, published *Beschreibung eines Augen-Spiegels*, which announced his invention of the ophthalmoscope and an explanation of its use. The introduction of the ophthalmoscope was the most significant advance in ophthalmology since the development of cataract surgery and marked the beginning of modern ophthalmology. This same year he advocated Young's *Three Components Theory* of color vision (1801), and it became accepted as the Young–Helmholtz theory of color perception.

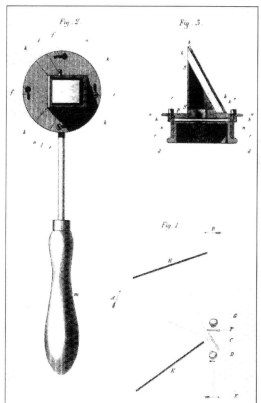

Illustration of the ophthalmoscope from *Beschreibung eines Augen-Spiegels* (1851) by Hermann von Helmholtz

1851   The Epkens ophthalmoscope was introduced. EPKENS, an instrument maker in Amsterdam who worked for Donders, replaced the glass plates with a mirror, the center of which did not have silvering.

1851   HENRY WILLARD WILLIAMS (1821–1895) of Harvard gave the first clinical course in ophthalmology in America.

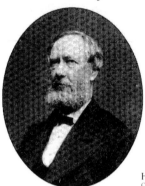

Henry Willard Williams (1821–1895)
Courtesy of Francis A. Countway Library of Medicine, Boston, MA

1851   AUGUSTIN PRICHARD (1818–1899), an ophthalmologist in Bristol, was the first to propose the enucleation of an injured eye for the prevention of sympathetic ophthalmia.

c. 1852   ADOLPHE HANNOVER developed an innovative way to cut thin sections for examinations under a microscope. The technique involved using chromic acid to harden the tissues before cutting.

1852   HENRY HAYNES WALTON of London published A practical treatise on the diseases of the eye in England and the United States. Walton was the founder of an eye clinic (1843) that evolved into the Central London Ophthalmic Hospital, which he served as director.

1852   SIR WILLIAM BOWMAN of London stressed the importance of digital estimation of ocular pressure and advocated its relief by surgical means.

1852   WILHELM AUGUST JOSEPH SCHLAGINWEIT (1792–1854) of Germany published Die bösartige Augenentzündung der Neugeborenen, which discussed the prevention and treatment of ophthalmia neonatorum. He asserts that prophylactic measures are the only sure way to deal with ophthalmia neonatorum. Schlaginweit suggests appropriate regulations for midwives, emphasizing the importance of cleanliness. Once the disease is contracted, he prescribes cleaning of the affected eyes as a curative procedure.

1852   HERMANN VON HELMHOLTZ in Königsberg described modifications of his ophthalmoscope designed by his machinist E. REKOSS to allow a clear focusing of the image on the observer's retina. Rekoss's improvement consisted of two rotatable disks containing lenses. The Rekoss disk has been incorporated in hand ophthalmoscopes since that time.

1852   *The pathology of the human eye* by JOHN DALRYMPLE, demonstrator of pathology in the Saunderion Institution of Moorfields Hospital, was published shortly after the author's death. Dalrymple shared the widely held prejudice against drawing conclusions on the basis of microscopic observations.

1852   CHRISTIAN GEORG RUETE, now director of the eye clinic at Leipzig, introduced indirect ophthalmoscopy. The instrument he described in his monograph *Der Augenspiegel und des Optometer für practische Aerzte* was essentially the same instrument proposed by Charles Babbage in 1847 and disparaged by Wharton Jones. Ruete introduced a practical lens system for examining the inverted image and also improved the illumination.

1852   THEODOR BILHARZ (1825–1862) of Cairo, known in ophthalmology for his studies of trachoma, discovered *Schistosoma haematobium*.

1852–1859   *Iconographic ophtalmologique*, the masterpiece of JULES SICHEL of Paris, was published.

1853   LORD JOSEPH LISTER (1827–1912) after graduating in medicine from the University of London published 'Observations on the contractile tissue of the iris.' He showed that the contractile tissue of the iris consisted of smooth muscle, the first correct account of the mechanism of dilating the pupil.

1853   ANTOINE CRAMER (1822–1855) of Holland published *Physiologische Abhandlung über das Accomodations-Vermögen der Augen*. This valuable essay explains the accommodation process in the eye, concluding that the lens increases convexity in accommodation. Cramer also designed an improved ophthalmoscope.

1853   ADRIEN CHRISTOPHE VAN TRIGT (1825–1864), at the University of Utrecht, published his classic dissertation on the ophthalmoscope, *De oogspiegel*. It included the earliest popular ocular fundus drawings.

1853   HENRI AUGUST SERRE (1802–1870) of Alais, France published *Essai sur les phosphènes*, a comprehensive summary of his work on phosphenes. Phosphenes, the luminous impressions seen when pressure is put on the eye, were used to diagnose various visual defects before the invention of the ophthalmoscope and remain an interesting method for ascertaining the function of the retina.

1853   ERNST ADOLF COCCIUS (1825–1890), an ophthalmology professor at the University of Leipzig, published *Ueber die Anwendung des Augen-*

Spiegels nebst Angabe eines neuen Instrumentes. Coccius describes his adaptation of the Helmholtz ophthalmoscope for use in either direct or indirect ophthalmoscopy, making use of a convex lens and a mirror. With his improved instrument, Coccius gave the first report of retinal tears associated with retinal detachment. In addition, he was the first to describe the reflex of the fovea centralis.

1853   The French ophthalmology journal, *Archives d'Opthalmologie*, began publication. Despite a hiatus in 1854, the journal continues to be published to the present time.

1853   ALBRECHT VON GRAEFE of Berlin began advocating tenotomies for the treatment of strabismus and devised a muscle hook to facilitate performing them.

1853   SIR WILLIAM BOWMAN at Moorfields described a new procedure for lacrimal obstruction. He slit the canaliculus and passed probes devised for that purpose through the canal and into the nose.

1853   The term 'ophthalmoscope' was introduced into the literature in its modern sense as the title of a paper by MARESSAL DE MARSILLY of Calais France in the *Annales d'Oculistique*. The instrument had previously been called an eye mirror or eye speculum.

1853   JEAN JULIEN VAN ROOSBROECK, professor of ophthalmology at Ghent, published *Cours d'ophthalmologie*, the first major systematic textbook of ophthalmology written by a Belgian. It was noted for its excellent chapter on contagious ophthalmias.

1853   JEAN-NICOLAS DEMARQUAY (1814–1875) published *Des tumeurs de l'orbite*, one of the earliest works on orbital tumors. This was followed in 1860 by a more extensive work *Traité des tumeurs de l'orbite*.

1854   CARSTEN HOLTHOUSE (1810–1890), a London surgeon, published *Six lectures on the pathology of strabismus and its treatment by operation*. He discusses the anatomy and physiology of the eye muscles, varieties of strabismus, their causes and diagnoses, operations to cure squint and reasons for their failures.

1854   CARL WEDL (1815–1891) was appointed professor of histology at the University of Vienna, where he was an important early contributor to ophthalmic histology and pathology. He was among the first to apply the cell theory to ocular pathology.

1854   ISAAC HAYS (1796–1879) of Philadelphia edited the American edition of Lawrence's text, *On diseases of the eye*. Hayes reported on the successful use of McAllister's cylindrical lenses to correct astigmatisms. This was one of the earliest American reports of astigmatism. Hays also served as editor to the *American Journal of the*

Medical Sciences (1826–1879), which carried numerous case reports of eye diseases.

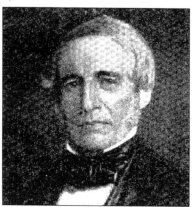

Isaac Hays
(1796–1879)

1854   ADOLPHE HANNOVER of Copenhagen proposed a radial sector conceptualization of the vitreous, with sections arranged around a central core area, similar to the sections of a cross-sectioned orange. Later authors adopted aspects of this and the lamellar theory to argue that the center of the vitreous contained sections while the exterior was made of layers.

1854   ELKANAH WILLIAMS (1822–1888) of Cincinnati published two articles on the ophthalmoscope, describing the view seen in a normal eye as well as abnormalities of the fundus, including retinal detachment.

1854   KARL WILHELM VON ZEHENDER (1819–1916), a student of Jaeger and von Graefe, modified the ophthalmoscope by adding a convex mirror.

1854   ANDREAS ANAGNOSTAKIS (1826–1897) was appointed director of the Ophthalmiatric Institute in Athens and published *Essai sur l'exploration de la rétine et des milieux de l'oeil sur le vivant, au moyen d'un nouvel ophthalmoscope*. It described the invention of a simplified ophthalmoscope that uses only a perforated concave mirror. This is the first work in French on the ophthalmoscope.

1854   EDUARD JAEGER (1818–1884), lecturer in ophthalmology at the University of Vienna, designed an improved ophthalmoscope, which he used to make drawing of the fundus requiring 40 to 120 hours for each illustration. Jaeger also invented an apparatus that calculated ocular refraction using the principle of the ophthalmoscope. The same year he was the first to publish a description and picture of the glaucomatous disc, but he incorrectly depicted the disc as swelling of the papillary tissues. He also was the first to describe the fundus changes of diabetes. Finally in 1854 Jaeger published *Über Staar und Staaroperationen*, providing a description of the pathological states of the lens based upon ophthalmoscopic examinations.

1854   GEORG MEISSNER (1829–1905), an anatomist and physiologist at Göttingen, published *Beiträge zue Physiologie des Sehorgans* in which he described the measurement of torsional movements of the eye.

1854   The anatomist PIERRE GRATIOLET used dissection material to support his claim that fibers of the optic tract pass beyond the thalamus into the occipital and parietal cortices.

1854   *Archiv für Ophthalmologie* was founded by ALBRECHT VON GRAEFE. From its inception von Graefe published his most significant articles in this journal, including his finding of the von Graefe sign in exophthalmic goiter. The same year von Graefe also noted pulsating vessels at the optic disc in patients with severe glaucoma.

1854   HERMANN VON HELMHOLTZ at Königsberg designed the modern ophthalmometer or keratometer. He modified one of the types of heliometers and produced an instrument that consisted of a telescope having in front of its objective two plates of glass with parallel plane surfaces placed side by side. By rotating the plates, the two images are separated and the amount of displacement of the images can be calculated by the angle made by the plates with the axis of the telescope.

1854–1860   CHRISTIAN RUETE, professor of ophthalmology at Leipzig, published his six-volume atlas and text, *Bildliche Darstellung der Krankheiten des menschlichen Auges*. This was an important work on eye diseases, therapeutics, ocular surgery, and gross pathology.

1855   CHARLES PIERRE DENONVILLIERS (1808–1872), a professor at the University of Paris, published *Traité théorique et pratique des maladies des yeux*. The topics covered include diseases of the eye, orbit, tear ducts, eyebrows, and eyelids.

1855   HENRY HANCOCK (1809–1880) of London published *On the ophthalmia of children or remittent ophthalmia*. Hancock served at the Royal Westminster Ophthalmic Hospital and the Charing Cross Hospital Medical School and devised a procedure known as the division of the ciliary muscle for glaucoma.

1855   RICHARD L. LIEBREICH (1830–1917) designed a tubular ophthalmoscope that could be combined with a camera lucida in the tube at the observer's end to permit the projection of an image of the fundus. This permitted the projected image to be drawn or projected onto a photographically sensitive glass plate for fundus photography. The drawings Liebreich accumulated served as the basis for his 1863 atlas, the first atlas of ophthalmoscopy.

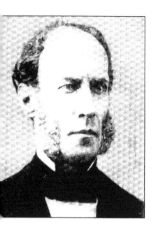

Eduard Jaeger
(1818–1884)

Illustration from *über Staar
and Staaroperationen* (1854)
by Eduard Jaeger

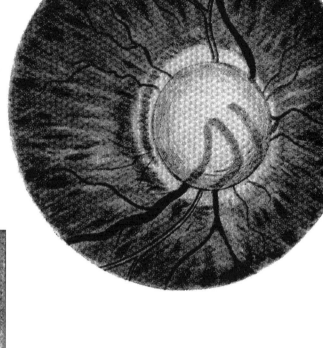

George Critchett
(1817–1882)

1855	BARTOLOMEO PANIZZA, professor of anatomy in Pavia, localized visual function to the posterior cortex of the brain. This conclusion was drawn from postmortem human material and experimentally induced lesions in dog brains.
1855	GEORGE CRITCHETT (1817–1882), a renowned English ophthalmic surgeon, published *Practical remarks on strabismus with some novel suggestions respecting the operation.* He describes his surgery procedure for strabismus using a subconjunctival technique and described an advancement procedure. In the same year Critchett published *Original observations founded upon a series of cases of extirpation of the globe,* which improved the enucleation procedure.
1855	EDWIN CANTON (1817–1885), a Charing Cross Hospital lecturer, published *Surgical and pathological observations.* It includes one of the most complete descriptions of intraocular and subconjuctival cysticercus infection.
1855	GEORGE WILSON (1818–1859) used statistical analyses in his *Researches on colour-blindness with a supplement on the danger attending the present system of railway and marine coloured signals,* to show that about 5.6% of the general population was color-blind. He highlighted the inherent dangers involved in the current color-based signals for railroad, marine, and military systems. In the same year he developed a technique for testing color blindness by using different colored 'worsteds.' Wilson was the first Englishman to urge screening of railway and military personnel for color blindness.
1855	ADOLF WEBER (1829–1915) began his practice in Darmstadt, Germany, and recorded an early observation of glaucomatous cupping. He subsequently published a number of important observations regarding the causes and treatment of glaucoma.

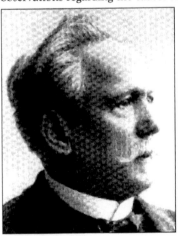

Adolf Weber
(1829–1915)

1855   EDUARD JAEGER in Vienna published *Beiträge zur Pathologie des Auges* that included his fundus paintings. The illustrations were instrumental in educating ophthalmologists as to the fundus appearance in such diseases as retinitis pigmentosa, glaucoma, diabetes, and choroidal melanoma.

1855   ALBRECHT VON GRAEFE of Berlin gave his landmark description of 'excavation of the nerve head' seen in advanced glaucoma with the ophthalmoscope.

1855   RICHARD L. LIEBREICH in Paris described 'retinal apoplexy' caused by central vein thrombosis.

1855   HERMANN VON HELMHOLTZ, now in Bonn, published *Ueber das sehen des Menschen*, popular lectures on the eye as an optical instrument, the perception of light, and the sensation of sight.

1855–1858   In a series of articles published in *Archiv für Ophthalmologie*, ALBRECHT VON GRAEFE in Berlin explained the use of iridectomy for the treatment of iritis, irido-choroiditis, and glaucoma. Von Graefe's perfection of the latter operation revolutionized the treatment of acute glaucoma.

1855   JAMES DIXON (1813–1896), surgeon to Moorfields and St. Thomas' Hospital, published *A guide to the practical study of diseases of the eye*. This was an important work on the diseases of the eye in which healthy and diseased tissues are analyzed.

1856   WILHELM HIS (1831–1904) of Basel published his notable work *Beiträge zur normalen und pathologischen Histologie der Cornea*. He invented a microtome which was capable of producing serial sections.

1856   RUDOLF LUDWIG KARL VIRCHOW (1821–1902) was appointed professor of pathology and director of the Pathological Institute in Berlin. Following his appointment, Virchow announced his theory that the cell was the fundamental living unit in both health and disease.

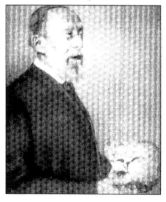

Rudolf Virchow
(1821–1902)

1856   ALBRECHT VON GRAEFE of Berlin described homonymous hemianopia, which in some cases he found associated with lesions in the cerebrum.

1856   CARL FERDINAND VON ARLT was appointed professor of ophthalmology at the University of Vienna. In the same year he reported that, on the basis of his dissections, myopia was the result of elongation of the globe.

1856   ROUGET in France described the fine structure of the uveal tract, including the ciliary muscle. This led the French to call it 'the muscle of Rouget,' while the Germans termed it 'the muscle of Müller.'

1856   HENRY WILLARD WILLIAMS published *On the treatment of iritis without mercury*. Williams fought against the use of mercury in the treatment of iritis because of its debilitating toxic effects and introduced the nonmercurial treatment of iritis.

1857   ANGE MARIE FRANÇOIS GUÉPIN (1805–1873) of France published *Études théoriques & cliniques sur les maladies des yeux*. An ardent socialist, Guépin was active in the revolutions of 1830 and 1848. His political views led to his dismissal from his position at the Hôtel Dieu, after which he continued to practice for some years, treating only the poor.

1857   CARL FRIEDRICH RICHARD FÖRSTER (1825–1902) in Breslau described his photometric apparatus and its use in the examination of healthy eyes and in cases of nightblindness in his *Über Hemeralopie und die Anwendung eines Photometers im Gebiete der Ophthalmologie*. He is

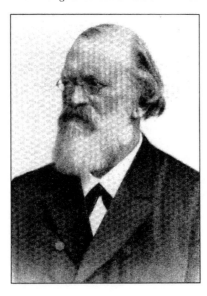

Carl Friedrich Richard Förster
(1825–1902)

considered to be the inventor of the photometer and the founder of ophthalmological photometry.

1857 ALBRECHT VON GRAEFE in Berlin invented a 'tenotomy hook' to facilitate strabismus surgery.

1857 JOHN FREMLYN STREATFEILD (1828–1886), a surgeon at Moorfields Hospital, described a technique for the grooving and sectioning of the tarsus for the treatment of cicatricial ectropion. He also described a partial exenteration technique involving removal of tarsi, conjunctival sac, and lid margins (ablation of the socket).

1857 SIR WILLIAM BOWMAN in London introduced the operation of canaliculotomy in preparation of probing or as a procedure for epiphora.

1857 The First International Ophthalmology Congress convened at Brussels in September with LOUIS SALOMON FALLOT of Belgium as its president. This is stated to be the first international medical congress of any sort to be held.

1857 CHRISTIAN GEORG RUETE followed Donders's technique and used afterimages to study ocular movements. Similar studies by Helmholtz (1863) and Hering (1868), among others, followed.

1858 FRIEDRICH PHILIPP RITTERICH, professor of ophthalmology at the University of Leipzig, published his text on eye surgery, *Lehre von den blutigen Augenoperationen am menschlichen Körper*. The excellent drawings show ophthalmological instruments, various phases of eye operations, and representations of eye diseases.

1858 JABEZ HOGG (1817–1899), ophthalmic surgeon to the Royal Westminster Ophthalmic Hospital among others, published *The ophthalmoscope; its mode of application explained*. The text includes cases of eyes examined by the ophthalmoscope and illustrations of the appearance of various diseases.

1858 ANTONIO QUAGLINO (1817–1894) of Milan was the author of the first ophthalmoscopic atlas published in Italy, *Sulle malattie interne dell'occhio*.

1858 RUDOLPH VIRCHOW in Berlin published *Die Cellular pathologie*, supporting his theory that all manifestations of disease can be traced to disturbances of living cells.

1858 THOMAS NUNNELEY (1890–1870), a surgeon at the Leeds Eye and Ear Infirmary, published *On the organs of vision: their anatomy and physiology*. It was a treatise on the laws of light, physiology of vision, and the structure of the human eye and its appendages.

1858 GEORGE CRITCHETT of Moorfields modified Bowman's

canaliculotomy procedure for epiphora by adding the 'three-snip procedure.'

1858   HEINRICH MÜLLER of Würzburg noted on the basis of his pathologic studies that in certain cases of trauma to the eye, tractional vitreous bands caused retinal detachment.

1858   SIR WILLIAM BOWMAN of London modified Anel and Petit's techniques for lacrimal probing of the nasolacrimal duct by slitting the lower canaliculus and dilating the nasolacrimal duct through the canaliculus by means of increasingly larger probes.

1858   EDWARD HARTSHORNE (1818–1885), a surgeon at the Wills Hospital in Philadelphia, edited an American edition of T. Wharton Jones's *Principles and practice of ophthalmic surgery*. Hartshorne played a prominent role in the development of ophthalmology in Philadelphia.

1858   ADOLF WEBER of Darmstadt reported a treatment for lens removal in high myopia. This operation was subsequently pursued and reported on by him in 1885.

1858   CASIMIR SPERINO of Turin published an important paper using meaningful statistics to demonstrate the superiority of intracapsular cataract extraction over other techniques.

1859   ADOLF ZANDER (d. 1863) of Chemnitz, Germany published the first comprehensive textbook on ophthalmoscopy, *Der Augenspiegel*. Zander's book provides a history of the ophthalmoscope, describes the various types of ophthalmoscopes, gives guidelines for its use, and describes the appearance of the normal fundus oculi and its appearance in various pathologic conditions. A second englarged edition appeared in 1862.

1859   SAMUEL DAVID GROSS (1805–1884), professor of surgery at Jefferson Medical College, published *A system of surgery*. His work included several chapters on the eye and was the source of instruction for American general surgeons who did most of the eye surgery in this country.

1859   FRANÇOIS ANTHIME EUGÈNE FOLLIN (1823–1867), professor of surgery at the University of Paris, published *Leçons sur l'application de l'ophthalmoloscope au diagnostic des maladies de l'oeil*.

1859   RICHARD L. LIEBREICH in Paris gave a detailed description of the fundus changes in nephritis.

1859   HERMANN JAKOB KNAPP (1832–1911) published *Die Krümmung der Hornhaut des menschlichen Auges*, a valuable monograph on the curvature of the cornea.

1859   JOHN WHITAKER HULKE (1830–1895), on the staff at Moorfields, published *The morbid changes in the retina as seen in the eye of the living person and after removal from the body.* He provided microscopic correlations to some of the new discoveries made with the ophthalmoscope.

1859   SIR JOHN FREDERICK WILLIAM HERSCHEL (1792–1871), the English astronomer and physicist, having accepted Young's concept of three primary colors, coined the term 'trichromic' to describe normal vision and 'dichromic vision' to describe those who can only see the colors blue and yellow.

1859   WILLIAM WHITE COOPER published *On wounds and injuries of the eye*, the first text to be devoted entirely to injuries of the eye. This text refined and popularized Victor Stoeber's method of enucleation.

1859   In Italy, the Casati Law was passed, regulating the practice of medicine. It required that every university medical school establish at least one eye department.

1859   At the Heidelberg Congress, FRANS CORNELIS DONDERS coined the term 'hypermetropia' and differentiated it from presbyopia. Donders also coined the terms refraction, emmetropia, ametropia, and aphakia—key words in the language of refraction.

c. 1860   CARL LUDWIG WILHELM BRUCH (1819–1884) noted the 'tapetum of mammals and the structureless membrane' which was named Bruch's membrane.

1860   SILAS WEIR MITCHELL (1829–1914), a Philadelphia neurologist, in his 'In the production of cataracts in frogs by the administration of sugar,' recognized that diabetic cataracts were the result of elevated blood sugar. This appears to be the first published ophthalmic research done in the United States.

1860   JOSEF PILZ (1818–1866) of Prague, the state ophthalmologist for the Kingdom of Bohemia, published *Compendium der operativen Augenheilkunde*. This was the first book to contain a topographic anatomy of the human eye. This is followed by a discussion of the types of wounds and wound healing occurring with surgery. Next is a description of the various operations, including personal comments and experiences.

1860   JAMES CLERK MAXWELL (1831–1879), at King's College, London, invented a colorimeter that measured color matching and light intensity.

1860   JOHN WILHELM OGLE, a neurologist at St. George's Hospital, London, promoted the use of the ophthalmoscope in detecting cerebral disease. He presented this idea in an article in the *Medical Times*.

1860   SIR JONATHAN HUTCHINSON (1828–1913) of London, a renowned surgical pathologist, ophthalmologist, and dermatologist, was the first to give a histological description of basal cell carcinoma.

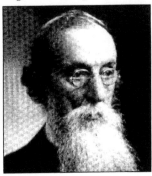

Sir Jonathan Hutchinson
(1828–1913)

1860   SIR WILLIAM BOWMAN described the 'antiglaucoma iridectomy,' which he erroneously believed restored communication between the vitreous and anterior chamber.

1860   ELKANAH WILLIAMS was appointed to the newly established chair at Miami (Ohio) Medical College and delivered a course of didactic lectures on ophthalmology during that year.

1860–1861   KARL STELLWAG VON CARION (1823–1904), professor of ophthalmology in Vienna, and CARL WEDL, professor of histology in Vienna, published *Atlas der pathologischen Histologie des Auges*. This was the first histologic pathology atlas of the eye. The atlas was the result of ten years of work.

1861   JOHN WHITAKER HULKE of Moorfields published *A practical treatise on the use of the ophthalmoscope*. He discussed the theory of the ophthalmoscope, a description of various ophthalmoscopes, and an account of progress made in ophthalmoscopic diagnosis between 1859 and 1861.

1861   GIACOBBE RAVÀ (1837–1911), ophthalmology professor at Pavia, revived the ancient procedure of coloring corneal opacities.

1861   BERNHARD RUDOLPH KONRAD VON LANGENBECK, the premier German clinical surgeon and teacher of his time, founded the *Archiv für klinische Chirurgie* in which many important articles relevant to eye surgery appeared.

1861   GEORGE CUVIER HARLAN (1835–1909), a major figure in the 'Philadelphia School of Ophthalmology,' was appointed attending surgeon at the Wills Eye Hospital. Among his many contributions to the field were his invention of the malingering test, the formulation of affixed bifocal segment spectacle lens, and his operation for symblepheron.

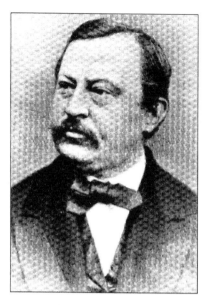

Karl Stellwag von Carion
(1823–1904)

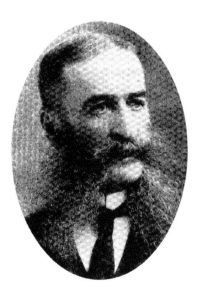

George Cuvier Harlan
(1835–1909)

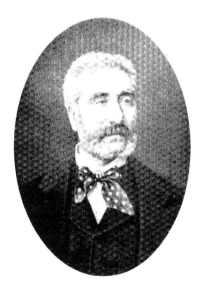

Marc Giraud-Teulon
(1816–1887)

1861   SIR JONATHAN HUTCHINSON reported that interstitial keratitis is a symptom of congenital syphilis. Interstitial keratitis, notched teeth, and labyrinth disease, which he describes as three major findings in congenital syphilis, became known as the 'Hutchinson triad.'

1861   MARC GIRAUD-TEULON (1816–1887) of Paris designed a binocular ophthalmoscope and explained its basic principles. The instrument used prisms as reflectors and was held by the examiner in one hand close to his or her eyes. It produced a small inverted image.

1862   HASKET DERBY (1835–1914) began his practice of ophthalmology in Boston after four years of study in Europe. A surgeon at the Massachusetts Charitable Eye and Ear Infirmary for 30 years and one of the founders of the American Ophthalmological Society, he wrote extensively on cataract surgery and was a pioneer in the use of anesthesia in this operation.

1862   CHARLES DEVAL of Paris published *Traité théorique et practique des maladies des yeux*. This was Deval's final work and represents 20 years of ophthalmologic practice and the examination of more than 20,000 pairs of eyes.

1862   THOMAS WHARTON JONES, in London, distinguished the disease scleritis from conjunctivitis, demonstrating that the inflammation in scleritis was independent of the conjunctiva.

1862   HERMANN SNELLEN (1834–1908) of Utrecht introduced the Snellen test-types with the publication of his *Optotypi*. In the same year he developed a treatment for mild ectropion involving the use of full-thickness sutures to reappose the lower lid against the globe.

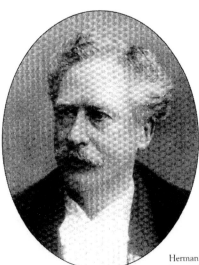

Hermann Snellen (1834–1908)
Courtesy of Francis A. Countway Library of Medicine, Boston, MA

1862	The *American Journal of Ophthalmology*, the first American journal of ophthalmology, was established by the controversial JULIUS HOMBERGER. He used the journal for self-promotion and two years later the *Journal* folded. In 1884, another journal appeared under the same name and continues to be published to the present time.
1862	CASIMIR SPERINO of Turin published *Études cliniques sur l'evactuation de l'humeur aquese dans les maladies de l'oeil* advocating the repeated evacuation of many eye diseases, including chronic glaucoma. He contended this treatment could also clear a cataract.
1863	ALBRECHT VON GRAEFE of Berlin initiated attempts at vitreous surgery with his report of cutting a posterior vitreous membrane by introducing a knife-needle into the vitreous through the pars plana. In the same year, von Graefe described a ptosis procedure consisting of undermining the skin of the upper lid and excising preseptal orbicularis muscle, and experimented with treating retinal detachment with subretinal fluid drainage through a posterior scleral puncture, but this failed to provide a permanent cure.
1863	ALBRECHT VON GRAEFE, ARLT, DONDERS, HESS, HORNER, and ZEHENDER founded the *Klinische Monatsblätter fur Augenheilkunde*. This journal continues to be published to the present day.
1863	DOUGLAS ARGYLL ROBERTSON (1837–1909) of Edinburgh, while looking for an agent to contract atropinized pupils, recognized the calabar bean as a useful drug in ophthalmology and published *The calabar bean as a new agent in ophthalmic medicine*.
1863	JULIUS JACOBSON, professor of ophthalmology at Königsberg, published *Ein neues und gefahrlos Operations-Verfahren zur Heilung des grauen Staares* that described Jacobsen's peripheral incision in cataract surgery. This was an important improvement in the cataract extraction operation.
1863	RICHARD LIEBREICH, practicing in Paris, published the first ophthalmoscopy atlas, *Atlas der Ophthalmoscopie*, illustrated with reproductions of his own fundus paintings. This was a model for all later atlases.
1863	JOHN HUGHLINGS JACKSON (1834–1911) of Yorkshire, a world-famous neurologist, promoted the ophthalmoscope in the *British Medical Journal* and elsewhere as a tool for identifying brain disease. He was an original member of the Ophthalmological Society.
1863	EDUARD ZEIS of Dresden published *Die Literatur und Geshichiste der Plastichen Chirurgie*. This, together with his *Handbuch der Plastichen Chirurgie*, continued to define the terms and scope of the new field of plastic surgery.

1863	The Heidelberg Ophthamological Society was founded by ALBRECHT VON GRAEFE and colleagues. This was one of the first local ophthalmological societies to be organized.
1863	ADOLF WEBER of Darmstadt modified Bowman's canaliculotomy method by slitting the upper canaliculus and dilating the lacrimal duct with a thick Bowman probe and sometimes fracturing the bony canal.
1863	ISABEL HAYES CHAPIN BARROWS (1845–1913), the first woman to practice ophthalmology in the United States, began studying medicine in India following the death of her husband. She returned to the United States to study medicine in Dansville, New York, where she was considered something 'radical.'

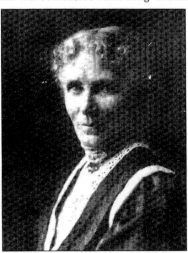

Isabel Hayes Chapin Barrows
(1845–1913)

1864	ROBERT BRUDENELL CARTER (1828–1918) of Nottingham, one of the first English physicians to use the ophthalmoscope, published an English translation of Zander's *Der Augenspiegel*.
1864	SILAS WIER MITCHELL, a Philadelphia neurologist, described in Civil War soldiers with neck wounds what is now called 'Horner's syndrome.' This was five years before Horner's report appeared.
1864	JEAN HUBERT THIRY (1817–1896) of Brussels published his successful results of transmitting infection from the eye to the urethra. He took pus from a case of 'true ocular blennorrhea' of a man and introduced it into the urethra of a volunteer. After 48 hours there was severe inflammation of the urethra with purulent discharge. This confirmed John Vetch's similar experiment carried out in 1820.
1864	PETER DIRCK KEYSER (1835–1897) of Philadelphia published

Glaucoma: its symptoms, diagnosis, and treatment, one of the earliest American works devoted to this subject. Keyser also established the Eye and Ear Hospital in Philadelphia about this time.

1864   GUSTAVUS HARTRIDGE (1849–1923) of London, an authority on error of refraction, published his extremely popular text *Refraction on the eye*. It contained information for diagnosis and the prescription of eyeglasses

1864   FRANS CORNELIS DONDERS, professor of anatomy and physiology at Utrecht, named and defined hypermetropia, and convinced physicians of its existence and its treatment. He made clear its distinction from myopia. He also defined astigmatism, aphakia, and other anomalies of refraction and accommodation. This was presented in Donder's monumental work published that year entitled *On the anomalies of accommodation and refraction of the eye*.

1864   ALBRECHT VON GRAEFE of Berlin devised a new incision for cataract surgery that he called the 'peripheral linear approach.' The von Graefe incision was almost linear rather than semicircular and gained immediate popularity because of less gaping of the wound and reduced endophthalmitis. Von Graefe's procedure included an extracapsular cataract extraction.

1864   MAURICE H. COLLIS (1824–1869) of England published *On the diagnosis of cancer and tumors*. In it he advocated that extirpation of the periosteum be included in exenteration for infiltrative malignant tumors of the orbit.

1864   The American Ophthalmological Society was founded on June 7, by ophthalmologists from Boston, New York, and Philadelphia. EDWARD DELAFIELD served as the first chairman, and HENRY DRURY NOYES (1832–1900) was appointed secretary.

1864   The New York Ophthalmological Society was founded.

1865   JOHN ZACHARIAH LAURENCE and THOMAS WINDSOM founded the *Ophthalmic Review*, which ceased publication in 1867 but was revived in 1881.

c. 1865   GUSTAV PASSAVANT (1815–1893) of Frankfurt am Main introduced the use of the lateral approach to orbital surgery to remove an orbital aneurysm.

1865   JAMES VOSE SOLOMON (1817–1899), professor of ophthalmology in Birmingham, published *Tension of the eyeball; glaucoma, etc.* He discusses iridectomy at length and advocates reducing the surgical coloboma by partially covering it with a conjuctival flap (artificial pterygium). For actue glaucoma he recommends 'intraocular myotomy' by an incision immediately behind the limbus and parallel to it.

1865   The University of Zurich became the first to give coeducational access to medical studies, preceding other universities by 50 years. Seven women medical students were taught ophthalmology by JOHANN FRIEDRICH HORNER, a distinguished ophthalmologist who discovered herpes corneae and for whom Horner's syndrome is named.

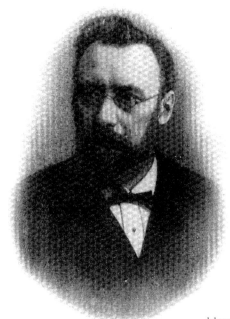

Johann Friedrich Horner
(1831–1886)

1865   F. BÖHMER of Würzburg described the use of alum hematoxylin to stain the nuclei of cells. This was an important milestone in the study of the histology of the eye and other organs.

1865   THEODOR LEBER (1840–1917) published a paper entitled 'The course and connections between the blood vessels in the human eye.' This was based on his adaptation of Ludwig's manometer to measure blood pressure and his own method of injecting vessels to trace the flow of fluids. Leber contributed greatly to the understanding of the ocular circulation.

1865   HENRY WILLARD WILLIAMS of Boston introduced the use of sutures to close the cataract wound. Williams used a pointed sewing needle and a strand of fine glover's silk. He placed a single suture at twelve o'clock through the flap.

1865   EZRA DYER (1836–1887) of Philadelphia reported that there was an important correlation between asthenopia and refractive errors. He was a pioneer in the study of the causes and treatment of eyestrain, and his methods of treatment became known as 'Dyerizing.'

1865   SIR JONATHAN HUTCHINSON of London reported on tobacco amblyopias in his article 'Cerebral amaurosis connected with the use of tobacco.' The article outlined the harmful ocular effects of tobacco.

1865   JOHN GREEN (1835–1913) of St. Louis formulated a test for identifying astigmatism that involved diagrams held 20 feet away.

1865–1866   ALARIK FRITHIOF HOLMGREN (1831–1897), physiologist at Uppsala, using a primitive galvanometer, demonstrated that the resting potential of the retina varied with exposure to light.

1866   MAX JOHANN SIGISMUND SCHULTZE (1825–1874), professor of anatomy at Bonn, published *Zur Anatomie und Physiologie der Retina*. This was an epoch-making histologic monograph on the nerve endings of the retina.

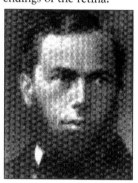

Max Johann Sigismund Schultze
(1825–1874)

1866   EUGÈNE BOUCHUT (1818–1891) of the Hôpital des Enfants Malades in Paris published *Du diagnostic des maladies du système nerveux par l'ophthalmoscopie*. This is an early work on the use of the ophthalmoscope in the diagnosis of diseases of the nervous system.

1866   WILLIAM WALLACE MCCLURE (1842–1923), a Philadelphia ophthalmologist, commenced a course of lectures on ophthalmology at the Wills Eye Hospital, one of the earliest systematic courses in Philadelphia.

1866   HENRY VEALE, a Scottish physician, coined the term 'rubella' for the viral infection also known as German measles. This disease, which can seriously affect the eye, was confused at the time with measles and smallpox.

1866	SALVIDOR FANO (1824–1895) at the University of Paris published *Traite practique des maladies des yeux*. In cases of retinal detachment, Fano advocated draining subretinal fluid through a scleral puncture and injecting an iodine solution in order to produce a 'chemically induced adhesive inflammatory response.'
1866	ALEXANDER PAGENSTECHER of Wiesbaden published his monograph on the advantages of extracting the cataractous lens within the unbroken capsule. Alexander, together with his younger brother and partner HERMANN (1844–1932), attained a reputation for surgical skill that attracted students and patients from all over Europe. They repopularized the intracapusular technique.
1866	NOTTIDGE CHARLES MACNAMARA (1832–1918), professor of ophthalmic surgery at Calcutta Medical College and later surgeon at the Royal Westminster Ophthalmic Hospital, published *Lectures on diseases of the eye*. This served as the basis for his later tome *A manual for diseases of the eye*. Macnamara was particularly noted as a cataract surgeon.
1866–1880	ERNST ABBE (1840–1905), working for Carl Zeiss, developed the substage condenser and oil immersion lenses for the microscope.
1867	ALBERT MOOREN of Düsseldorf published his major work *Ophthalmiatrische Beobachtungen*.
1867	The government in Bern established a 20-bed eye clinic in a house previously assigned to the state apothecary. HENRI DOR (1834–1912) was appointed director of the eye clinic and professor of ophthalmology. Dor contributed a number of papers on myopia, retinal detachment, color vision, color blindness, and tonometry.
1867	FRANCESCO MAGNI (1825–1887), professor of ophthalmology at the university in Bologna (1863), published *Lezioni teoriche di oftalmajatria*. A notable ophthalmic surgeon, Magni published numerous papers on cataract, glaucoma, keratitis, choroiditis, entropion, and central scotoma.
1867	ALBRECHT VON GRAEFE of Berlin published *Symptomenlehre der Augenmuskallähmungen*. This, presented on the occasion of his inauguration as professor at the University of Berlin, forms the basis of modern knowledge of the subject. It described conditions that can result from injuries to the eye muscles and methods of diagnosis to determine the extent of injury. Von Graefe presented the first thorough account of paralysis of the eye muscles. Laws of physiology that govern eye movements and the effects of impaired function in each of the ocular muscles were detailed.
1867	HERMANN VON HELMHOLTZ, now at Heidelberg, published *Handbuch*

Illustration of 'Hutchinson's teeth' of congenital syphilis from *Lectures on diseases of the eye* (1866) by Nottidge Charles Macnamara

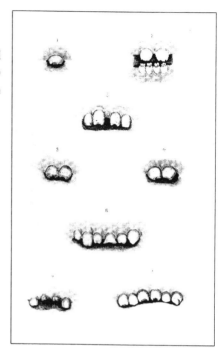

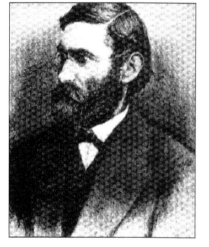

Ernst Abbe
(1840–1905)

Illustration of test-type from *Lectures on diseases of the eye* (1866) by Nottidge Charles Macnamara

129

der physiologischen Optik. This is one of the greatest works on physiologic optics. It included the author's detailed treatment of the dioptrics of the eye, his theory of accommodation, a description of the ophthalmoscope, an extended defense of the theory of visual perception, and a revival of Thomas Young's theory of color vision.

1867   LORD JOSEPH LISTER, professor of surgery at the University of Glasgow, wrote of his use of antiseptic principles in surgery in his article 'On the antiseptic principle in the practice of surgery.' This was in response to the high rates of infection following cataract and other surgery. Lister's introduction of antiseptic principles led to sterile ophthalmic surgery.

1867   GEORGE LAWSON (1831–1903) of Moorfields published *Injuries of the eye, orbit and eyelids*, describing the management of trauma to the eye ranging from superficial injuries to penetrating wounds and intraocular foreign bodies. In this same year, Lawson published a report of an exenteration procedure to eradicate an infiltrative malignant tumor of the orbit.

1867   LOUIS ÉMILE JAVAL (1839–1907) of Paris developed the astigmometer.

1867   NADEZHDA SUSLOVA, one of the pioneer women physicians of the Zurich Seven, presented her thesis on the lymphatic system in the human body and received the first medical degree given a woman by a recognized coeducational university with high academic standards.

1867   VICENZ CZERNY described his research on chorioretinal burns in animals caused by sunlight passed through a convex lens and a concave mirror.

1868   ABRAHAM METZ (1828–1876), ophthalmology professor at the Charity Hospital Medical College in Cleveland, published *The anatomy and histology of the human eye.* The book is distinguished by the bibliography, which contains titles published in Germany after 1857, indicating Metz's familiarity with current developments in his field.

1868   JEAN TIMOTHEE ÉMILE FOUCHER (1823–1867) taught ophthalmology at the University of Paris. His *Leçons sur la cataracte* was among the most important of his 141 publications, which also addressed deformities of the pupil, pterygium, entropion, and the use of glycerine in the treatment of trachoma.

1868   LUDWIG WILHELM MAUTHNER (1840–1894) of Vienna published *Lehrbuch der Ophthalmoscopie*, which discusses the discovery made with Helmholtz's ophthalmoscope and the methods of examiniation with this instrument. Mauthner was an authority on ophthalmoscopes.

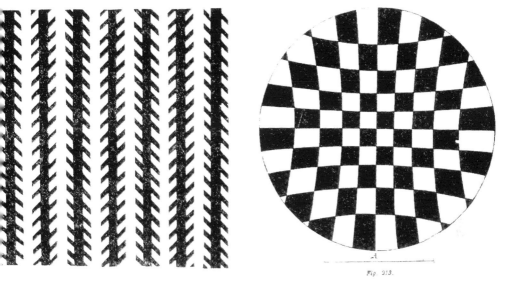

Fig. 213.

Illustrations of optical illusions from *Handbuch der physiologischen Optik* (1867) by Hermann von Helmholtz

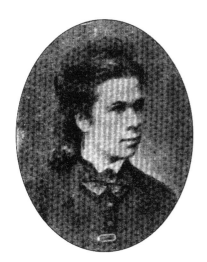

Nadezhda Suslova

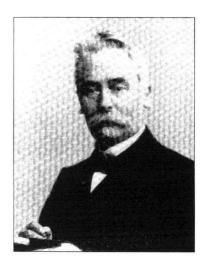

Albert Mooren
(1828–1899)

1868   CHARLES BADER (1825–1899), a German ophthalmologist who settled in London and practiced at Guy's Hospital, published *The natural and morbid changes of the human eye and their treatment*. The work covers ophthalmic developments in the treatment of disease for the previous 12 years, stressing the diagnostic use of the ophthalmoscope. Of note are the ten chromolithographic plates that show the eye as seen though an ophthalmoscope.

1868   CARL FRIEDRICH RICHARD FÖRSTER of Breslau invented the perimeter.

1868   HENRY POWER (1828–1911), a founding member of the Ophthalmological Society of the United Kingdom and its president for three years, published *Illustrations of some of the principal diseases of the eye*. It was an advanced book for the time, containing chapters on trauma, strabismus, and refractive and accommodative problems.

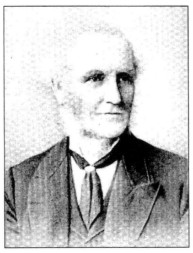

Henry Power
(1828–1911)

1868   HERMANN JAKOB KNAPP, professor at Heidelberg, immigrated to New York City, where he established the New York Ophthalmic and Aural Institute. Knapp also published *Die intraocularen Geschwülste*, which provided a thorough summary regarding the diagnosis and treatment of intraocular tumor.

1868   RUDOLF BERLIN (1833–1897) of Stuttgart popularized the removal of the lacrimal sac (dacryocystectomy) in place of slitting the canaliculus and introducing progressively larger probes.

1868   HENRY DRURY NOYES was appointed professor of ophthalmology and otology at the Bellevue Hospital Medical College. Noyes was among the first to investigate the retinopathy associated with glycosuria.

1868   KARL EWALD CONSTANTIN HERING (1834–1918), a professor of physiology in Vienna and an authority on the physiology of space perception, published *Die Lehre von binocularen Sehen*. Hering describes the principles of binocular vision and the function of the ocular muscles. Hering also discusses the relationship between accommodation and convergence.

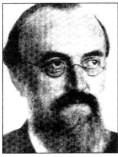

Karl Ewald Constantin Hering
(1834–1918)

1869–1870   JACOB HUGO GEROLD (1814–1898) of Aken, Germany published *Die ophthalmologische Physik und ihre Anwendung auf die Praxis*. This is a comprehensive survey of optics with strong sections on the making of glass and different kinds of spectacles, as well as the construction of optical instruments.

1869   HERMANN KNAPP, now at the New York Ophthalmic and Aural Institute, began the systematic reporting of his cataract operation results. His operation of choice evolved into an intracapsular extraction involving a tumbling procedure in which the lower equator of the lens is grasped, and by rotating the lens, this portion exits first through the wound. In the same year, Knapp of New York, collaborating with S. MOOS of Heidelberg, established the bilingual German and English *Archives of Ophthalmology and Otology*, which continues publication today as the *Archives of Ophthalmology*.

1869   THEODOR LEBER in Berlin demonstrated that the transparency of the

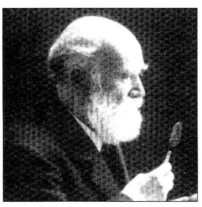

Theodor Leber
(1840–1917)

133

cornea is protected by the endothelium and that of the lens by its epithelium.

1869   JOHANN FRIEDRICH HORNER (1831–1836), professor of ophthalmology in Zurich, described the constellation of ptosis of the upper eyelid, elevation of the lower lid, enophthalmos, constriction of the pupil, narrowing of the palpebral fissure, anhidrosis, and flushing of the affected side of the face caused by paralysis of the cervical sympathetic nerves. This is commonly called Horner's syndrome.

1869   AUGUST RITTER VON REUSS (1841–1924), chief ophthalmologist at the Vienna Polyclinic and an authority on physiological optics, published *Ophthalmometrische Studien* in conjunction with M. WOINOW. Von Reuss contributed studies on the curvature of the cornea and myopia.

1869   EDUARD JAEGER of Vienna published *Ophthalmoskopischer Hand-Atlas*, one of the most important and widely used ophthalmoscopic atlases of the nineteenth century.

1869   SALOMON STRICKER (1834–1898), a Vienna pathologist, described the histology of the cornea in his *Versuche über Hornhautentz-undung*. He was a pioneer in the preparation of tissues for microscopy.

1869   DOUGLAS ARGYLL ROBERTSON, an ophthalmic surgeon to the Royal Infirmary at Edinburgh, described the abnormality of the pupil now known as the Argyll Robertson pupil.

1869   THEODOR ALBRECHT EDWIN KLEBS (1834–1913) described an improved method of embedding tissue in paraffin. This technique was soon adopted for ophthalmic histology and pathology.

1869   ALEXANDER IWANOFF (1836–1880), professor of ophthalmology at Kiev, observed that detachment of the vitreous often preceded retinal detachment and considered it a probable causative factor.

1869   JACQUES LOUIS REVERDIN (1842–1929), a Swiss surgeon, published his findings that an isolated piece of human epidermis would survive and grow when placed on a properly prepared bed, protected, and kept in contact with underlying and surrounding tissues.

1869   EDWARD GREELY LORING (1837–1888) of New York City described the first of his several improved models of the ophthalmoscope. The last version of the Loring ophthalmoscope was introduced in 1877 and gained great popularity in the United States. The instrument featured a mirror that could be tilted from side to side for examination of the right or left eye. In addition, it had a disk of 16 lenses with four supplementary lenses in the quadrant above.

1869   WILLIAM FISHER NORRIS (1839–1901) of Philadelphia, who had been studying ophthalmology in Europe, published his findings on the

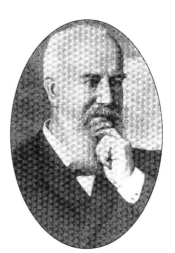

Louis de Wecker
(1832–1906)

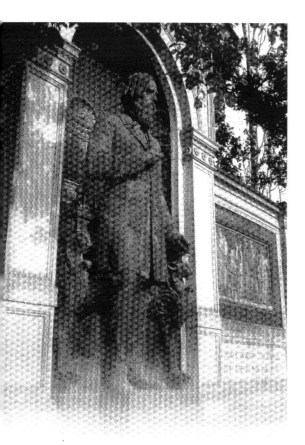

Albrecht von Graefe Monument, Berlin,
unveiled 1882

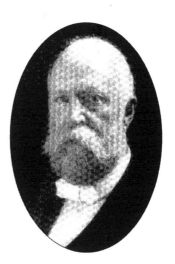

William Fisher Norris
(1839–1901)

histopathology of the cornea in an article entitled *Versuche über Hornhautentzundung* in conjunction with SALOMON STRICKER.

1869 The Manhattan Eye, Ear, Nose and Throat Hospital was founded by CORNELIUS REA AGNEW and DANIEL DE ROOSA (1838–1903).

1869 MAX BURCHARDT, ophthalmologist and dermatologist of Berlin, produced his international vision charts to determine visual acuity and visual range. These consisted of black discs photographically enlarged or reduced to obtain mathematically correct gradations of size.

1870 DOUGLAS ARGYLL ROBERTON, ophthalmic surgeon to the Royal Infirmary in Edinburgh, became one of the first ophthalmologists to accept Lister's antiseptic surgical techniques. Moorfields Eye Hospital soon followed, boiling instruments and treating them with carbolic acid. Their rate of surgical infections declined.

1870 ÉDOUARD MEYER (1838–1902) of Paris and HENRI DOR at Bern founded the *Revue Générale d'Ophtalmologie*.

1870 JULIUS VON SZYMANOWSKI (1829–1868), one of the leading surgeons of his day in Eastern Europe, modified Dieffenbach's ectropion surgery by adjusting the placement of the triangle. This resulted in 'lateral and superior support.' This was later called the Kuhnt–Szymanowski procedure.

1870 EMIL GRÜNING (1842–1914), an immigrant to the United States from Prussia, established his ophthalmology practice in New York and was chair of the eye department at Mount Sinai Medical Center. Grüning was among the first to show the detrimental effects of wood alcohol on the eye, and he designed a small hand magnet for the extraction of foreign bodies from the eye.

1870 LOUIS DE WECKER (1832–1906) of Paris and EDUARD JAEGER in Vienna, in their text *Traité des maladies du fond de l'oeil*, were the first to emphasize the frequent occurrence of retinal breaks in cases of spontaneous retinal detachment. They were also the first to postulate that liquid vitreous passing through retinal breaks was responsible for certain cases of detachment.

1870 GUSTAV SCHWALBE (1844–1916), the German anatomist, made the observation that when certain dyes were injected into the anterior chamber either in aqueous solution or in suspension, they promptly appeared in the veins on the surface of the globe. Schwalbe concluded that the anterior chamber was a lymphatic space in open communication with the anterior ciliary veins.

1870 THEODOR SAEMISCH (1833–1909), a graduate of the University of

Berlin, published *Das Ulcus corneae serpens und seine Therapie*. This provided the first full description of serpinginous ulcer of the cornea (Saemisch ulcer) and advocated its treatment by a procedure now known as the Saemisch incision.

1871   ANTONIO QUAGLINO, now professor of ophthalmology at Pavia, was the first to systematically employ sclerotomy for glaucoma. In the same year, he founded the journal *Annali di ottalmologia*.

1871   HENRY WILLARD WILLIAMS was appointed professor of ophthalmology at the Harvard Medical School.

1871   SIR THOMAS CLIFFORD ALLBUTT published *On the use of the ophthalmoscope in diseases of the nervous system and of the kidneys, also in certain other general disorders*. He described the effects of encephalic disease, such as epilepsy, chorea, and meningitis, upon the optic disk and retina, and advocated using the ophthalmoscope to diagnose and investigate neurological changes.

1871   JOHANN FRIEDRICH HORNER, professor of ophthalmology in Zurich, reported his discovery of herpes simplex of the cornea in the *Klinische Monatsblätter Augenheilkunde*.

1871   LEARTUS CONNOR (1843–1911) joined the faculty of the Detroit Medical College, subsequently becoming professor of diseases of the eye. He introduced a 'tucking' operation for the shortening of muscles in strabismus.

1871   ÉDOUARD MEYER of Paris published his remarkable *Traité des operation qui se pratiquent sur l'oeil*, the first surgical textbook of any type to contain series of photographs of actual operations. It contained close-up shots of strabismus, cataract, iridectomy, canthoplasty, and other surgery performed on cadavers. The photographer, DR. MONTMEJA, founded the first journal devoted to medical photography in 1869. Meyer also was the first ophthalmologist to attempt retinal suturing following sclerotomy in order to reattach the retina in retinal detachment.

1871   CORNELIUS REA AGNEW of New York described a new incision for drainage of the lacrimal sac made through the conjunctiva between the caruncle and the inner commissure of the eyelids.

1871   KARL ERNST THEODOR SCHWEIGGER (1830–1905) of Berlin published his *Handbuch der speciellen Augenheilkunde*, which contained both his teachings and those of von Graefe. This textbook was considered one of the most authoritative of the time.

1871   ISABEL HAYES CHAPIN BARROW purchased $100 worth of eye instruments and on May 29 opened her office at 628 F Street in

Washington for the practice of ophthalmology. She was the first woman with a formal medical education to practice ophthalmology in the United States.

1871   CARL WEIGERT (1845–1904) developed a method for staining paraffin and celloidin tissue sections. This technique was rapidly utilized in ocular pathology.

1871   PAUL JULIUS SCHRÖTER (1840–1930), an ophthlamologist in Leipzig, published his study of acquired nystagmus among miners.

1872   XAVIER GALEZOWSKI (1832–1907) founded the *Journal d'Ophtalmologie*, which in 1879 became the *Recueil d'Ophtalmologie*. He also published his major text *Traité des maladies des yeux* with good discussions of refraction and ophthalmoscopy.

1872   JOHN FREMLYN STREATFEILD at Moorsfield Hospital suggested in *The Lancet* removal of the tarsi, conjunctival sac, and lid margins (ablation of the socket) in some cases of enucleation.

1872   ALBRECHT NAGEL (1833–1895) of Germany established the *Janresbericht über Leistungen und Fortschritte im Gebiete der Ophthalmologie*. Nagel, an ophthalmology professor at Tübingen, was the author of several notable treatises on amaurosis and amblyopia, anomalies of refraction and accommodation, and binocular vision.

1872   HERMANN SCHMIDT-RIMPLER (1838–1915), professor of ophthalmology at Marburg, published his investigations on herpes of the cornea, confirming Horner's findings published the year before.

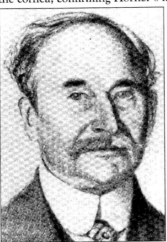

Hermann Schmidt-Rimpler
(1838–1915)

1872   OTTO HEINRICH ENOCH BECKER (1828–1890), a professor at the University of Heidelberg, published a compilation of all of the late Heinrich Müller's pioneering work on the anatomy, physiology, and pathology of the eye (*Gesammelte und hinterlassene Schriften*). Becker went on to formulate 'Becker's test' to diagnose astigmatism and 'Becker's sign,' which is the pulsation of retinal arteries.

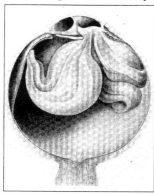

Illustration from *Atlas der pathologischen Topographie des Augues* (1874) by Otto Heinrich Enoch Becker

1872   The Madrid Ophthalmic Institute was opened by the Queen of Spain, and DELGADO JUGO (1830–1875) became its first director. He was a surgeon and teacher of distinction, and by translating De Wecker's text and Liebreich's atlas, he began the creation of a Spanish ophthalmic literature.

1872   LEON C. LE FORT (1829–1893) of Lille, France successfully used a full-thickness skin graft for the treatment of cicatricial ectropion.

1872   LÈOPOLD X. E. OLLIER (1830–1900), chief surgeon at the Hôtel Dieu de Lyon, reported the use of thin but relatively large 'split-thickness' skin grafts.

1873   GEORGE STRAWBRIDGE (1844–1914), a surgeon in the Civil War, was appointed lecturer in ophthalmology and otology at the University of Pennsylvania. In the same year, he published *Ophthalmic contribution*, which included his operation for the removal of iris cysts.

1873   RUDOLPH BERLIN of Stuttgart described the condition known as commotio retinae or Berlin's edema.

1873   HENRY DEWAR and JOHN GRAY MCKENDRICK, in Scotland, confirmed the work of Du Bois-Reymond and Holmgren, demonstrating that the resting potential of the retina varied with exposure to light.

1873   FERDINAND CUIGNET (b. 1823) introduced the 'shadow test' (retinoscopy or skiascopy) in examinations for astigmatism. It was widely employed first in England and then worldwide to examine patients.

1873   KARL ERNST THEODOR SCHWEIGGER, now professor at Göttingen, stated his theory that the cause of concomitant squint was the elastic predominance of one group of muscles over the opposing group.

1874–1880	ALFRED CARL GRAEFE (1830–1899) of Halle and THEODOR SAEMISCH of Bonn published *Handbuch der Gesamten Augenheilkunde*. This encyclopedic work attempted to summarize the new knowledge that had accumulated in ophthalmology during the preceding decades.
1874	MICHEL JULIEN MASSELON (1844–1917) of Paris, partner of LOUIS DE WECKER, began the publication of annual reports from their clinic entitled *Clinique ophthalmologique de Dr. de Wecker a Paris*.
1874	HERMANN JAKOB KNAPP of New York successfully completed the first transconjunctival orbitomy, removing a tumor of the optic nerve while preserving the eye.
1874	CARL FERDINAND VON ARLT, professor of ophthalmology in Vienna, perfected George Jäsche's blepharoplasty technique. The Jäsche–Arlt technique was still in use in the twentieth century, after further modification.
1874	HUBERT SATTLER (1844–1928) studied malignant tumors of the orbit and their treatment and published *Über die sogenannten Cylindrome*. In the same year, ROBERT SATTLER (1855–1939) published in the German literature a technique for exenteration based on that proposed by Collis in 1864.
1874	WILLIAM ALEXANDER MCKEOWN (1844–1904) of Ireland used a magnet to remove a foreign body from the vitreous and preserved a useful eye.
1874–1878	OTTO HEINRICH ENOCH BECKER, professor of ophthalmology at Heidelberg, issued his *Atlas der pathologischen Topographie des Auges* based on the study of 1800 specimens from the respected eye pathology laboratory at Heidelberg.
1875	OTTO HEINRICH ENOCH BECKER, professor of ophthalmology at Heidelberg, contributed his classical sections on the lens for the Graefe–Saemische *Handbuch*. This formed the basis for his later work *Zu Anatomie der gesunden und kranken Linse*.
1875	RICHARD CATON (1842–1926), a physician in Liverpool, demonstrated electrical differences in the posterior cortex following flashes of light.
1875	JOHN REISBERG WOLFE (1824–1904) of the Glasgow Ophthalmic Institute successfully repaired a defect of the lower eyelid using a full-thickness skin graft.
1875	CHRISTOPHER SMITH FENNER (1823–1879), a lecturer on eye disease at Louisville Medical College, wrote an early American work on physiologic optics and defects of the eye, *Vision: its optical defects and the adaption of spectacles*. It includes sections on the nature of light,

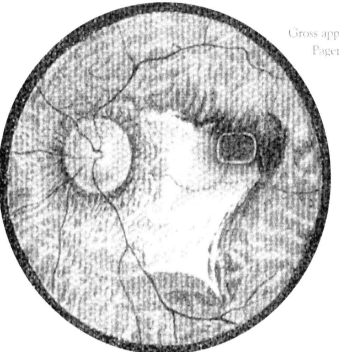

Gross appearance of choroiditis from
Pagenstecher and Genth (1875)

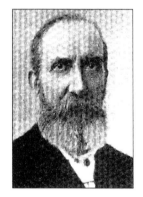

Hubert Sattler
(1844–1928)

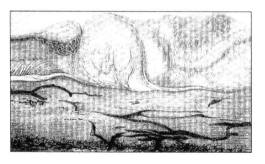

Microscopic appearance of choroiditis
from Pagenstecher and Genth (1875)

visual sensations and perceptions, and the treatment of errors of refraction and defects of accommodation.

1875   HERMANN PAGENSTECHER (1844–1932) of Wiesbaden and KARL PHILIPP GENTH (1844–1904) of Longenschwalbach published *Atlas of the pathological anatomy of the eyeball*. The specimens illustrated included 300 eyes collected by the authors and 500 additional eyes furnished by Sir William Bowman, Sir Johathan Hutchinson, Richard Liebreich, Edward Nettleship, and others.

1875   The Ophthalmological Congress at Heidelberg adopted a standardized system for lens grading based on their dioptric power. F. MONOYER (1836–1912) proposed the system at a previous meeting. This has been the worldwide standard since 1920.

1875   GEORGE WILSON'S prediction in his 1855 *Researches on colour-blindness* came true when two trains crashed in Sweden. ALARIK FRITHIOF HOLMGREN, the Swedish physiologist, demonstrated that the probable cause of the accidents was a missed color-based signal.

1875   ROBERT BRUDENELL CARTER of London published A *practical treatise on diseases of the eye*. His text covers the topics of ocular anatomy, examination pathology, physiology, and color sense.

1876   SILAS WEIR MITCHELL, a Philadelphia neurologist, introduced the term 'eyestrain' into the literature in his famous article 'Headaches from eyestrain' in the *American Journal of Medical Sciences*.

1876   FRANZ CHRISTIAN BOLL (1849–1879), professor of physiology in Rome, noted that the pigment described by Müller was bleached by light. He called the pigment 'Sehrot' (visual red).

1876   MAX KNIES (1851–1917), in Berlin, provided the first pathologic report on the condition of the chamber angle in glaucoma. Knies wrote in a paper in the *Archiv für Ophthalmologie*: 'The most important finding in genuine glaucoma is the circular adhesion of the iris periphery to the periphery of the cornea or the obliteration of the space of Fontana.'

1876   DAVID FERRIER in his important text *The functions of the brain* presented his studies regarding the stimulation and ablation of the occipital cortex.

1877   ADOLF KUSSMAUL of Strasbourg in his work on aphasia first used the term 'word-blindness' (*Worthblidheit*).

1877   RUDOLPH BERLIN of Stuttgart, a pioneer in comparative ophthalmology, described a retinal detachment in a horse, as well as an 'amaurotic cat's-eye' in another horse.

1877   WILHELM FRIEDRICH KÜHNE (1837–1900), professor of physiology at

Heidelberg University, published *Zur Photochemie der Netzhaut; Über der Sehpurpur*. This consisted of two of his papers on visual purple (rhodopsin).

1877   LUDWIG LAQUEUR (1838–1909), professor of ophthalmology at the University of Strasbourg, in an article entitled 'Über Atropin und Phisostrymin' reported 'a definite drop of elevated [intraocular] pressure after repeated installations of an 0.3% or 0.5% aqueous of physostigmine in five cases of glaucoma simplex and in one case of secondary glaucoma.' Laqueur himself was diagnosed with glaucoma in 1874.

1877   THEODOR LEBER, professor of ophthalmology in Göttingen, received the first Graefe Prize for a superior scientific paper. Leber provided a clear and comprehensive concept of aqueous formation and elimination. His landmark paper on this subject was published in the *Archiv für Ophthalmologie*.

1877   HENRI PARINAUD (1844–1905) of Paris published *Étude sur la névrite optique dans la meningite aiguë de l'enfance* on optic neuritis in childhood meningitis. Parinaud established a free eye clinic for the poor in Paris, which attracted students and practitioners from all over the world.

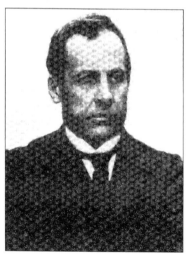

Henri Parinaud
(1844–1905)

1877   ALARIK FRITHJOF HOLMGREN of Uppsala devised a color blindness test using skeins of dyed wool to corroborate the Young–Helmholtz theory of color vision. He described this in a book in Swedish about color blindness in which he stressed the need to test railway and maritime employees. He also emphasized that the color-based signal system for trains and boats should be changed. An abbreviated English translation was published in the *Report of the Smithsonian Institute for 1877* entitled 'Theory and diagnosis of color blindness.'

1877   The first law preventing color-blind people from working on railroads was passed in Sweden. The work of HOLMGREN and GEORGE WILSON was instrumental in subsequently making color vision testing mandatory for railroad and marine employees.

1877   ADOLF WEBER of Berlin theorized that the cause of elevated intraocular pressure was 'a disturbance of outflow of 'lymph' in the anterior chamber angle' and not 'hypersecretion of aqueous,' as previously believed. He systematically studied the pressure-lowering effects of eserine and pilocarpine and strongly preferred the latter drug.

1877   WILLIAM FISHER NORRIS of Philadelphia, working with GEORGE A. PIERSOL at the University of Pennsylvania, continued his studies of the histology of the cornea, leading to the publication of their *Microscopical anatomy of the cornea.*

1877   According to the historian Burton Chance, VIGER published the first report describing methyl alcohol as a cause of blindness.

1877   STEIN, in Toronto, succeeded in taking a fundus photograph of a rabbit eye using Liebreich's stand ophthalmoscope.

1877   JAKOB STILLING (1842–1915) of Kassel, Germany, introduced a system of pseudoisochromatic plates for testing color vision.

1877   ROBERT BRUDENELL CARTER of London developed a photometer to test for color sense.

1877   ARTHUR VON HIPPEL (1841–1916) at Königsberg published his experiments with an improved keratoprosthesis. Despite the use of chloroform anesthesia, he was unable to achieve true clinical success with his device.

1878–1883   DAVID HAYES AGNEW (1818–1892) of Philadelphia published *The principles and practice of surgery, being a treatise on surgical diseases and injuries.* This includes a section on ocular anatomy, diseases, diagnosis, and medical surgical treatment. With SAMUEL D. GROSS's *A system of surgery* (1859), this was one of the most important books for American general surgeons who operated on the eye.

1878   OLIVER WENDELL HOLMES (1809–1894) of Boston was responsible for the publication of *Visions: A study of false sight* by EDWARD HAMMOND CLARKE (1820–1877) the late professor of materia medica at Harvard. The book discusses the neuropsychiatric aspects of visual illusions and hallucinations in those about to die.

1878   Ophthalmology and otolaryngology were acknowledged as legitimate subspecialties by the American Medical Association by permitting the establishment of the AMA Section on Ophthalmology, Otology, and Laryngology.

1878   KARL EWALD CONSTANTIN HERING, a professor of physiology at the University of Prague, published his theory of color vision in *Zur Lehre von Lichtsinne*. In opposition to Young's theory, Hering believed that complementary colors were the result of opposing retinal stimulation.

1878   CHARLES A. SPENCER succeeded in making the first optical-quality glass produced in the United States, for which he won a gold medal at the Paris Exposition of 1878.

1878   JOSEPH PRIESTLEY SMITH (1845–1933), an ophthalmic surgeon in Birmingham, was awarded the Jacksonian prize of the Royal College of Surgeons for his essay 'Glaucoma: its causes, symptoms, pathology and treatment.' This was published the following year and was considered the most authoritative English textbook on glaucoma of its time.

1879   HERMANN MUNK in his classic paper 'Physiologie der Sehsphäre der Grosshirnrinde' presented the detailed anatomy of the decussation of the optic chiasm.

1879   ERNST PFLÜGER (1846–1903) became professor of ophthalmology at Bern. Pflüger's studies covered many ophthalmic subjects, but his most notable achievements included inventing a refraction ophthalmoscope and his studies on skiascopy, intraocular circulation, glaucoma, and anomalies of refraction.

1879   The physiologist MATHIAS DUVAL (1844–1907) introduced an improved method of tissue embedding using collodion.

1879   ALBERT NEISSER (1855–1916), a dermatologist at Breslau, by using recently introduced bacteriological techniques, discovered that the gonococcus was the specific organism responsible for ophthalmia of the newborn (ophthalmia neonatorum).

1879   THEODOR LEBER of Göttingen isolated the fungus *Aspergillus glaucus* from corneal ulcers and then artificially caused the disease in animals, thus demonstrating fungi could cause keratitis.

1879   SIR WILLIAM RICHARD GOWERS (1845–1915) of Queen Square in London published *A manual and atlas of medical ophthalmoscopy*. Gowers stresses the value of the ophthalmoscope in diagnosis and includes his own original observations. Although he was primarily a neurologist, his writings and illustrations had a profound impact on ophthalmology.

1879   FRIEDRICH SIGMUND MERKEL (1857–1919) and SHIEFFERDECKER in Germany introduced the use of a commercial variant of collodion called celloidin for embedding tissues.

1880   IGNATZ VON PECZELY of Hungary published *Discoveries in the realm of nature and the art of healing* that gave the first mention of iridology.

1880   LOUIS BRAILLE (1809–1892) described his invention of a system of writing and printing for the blind. Braille, himself blind from sympathetic ophthalmia resulting from an accident at age three, attended and taught at the Institution Nationale des Jeunes Aveugles in Paris.

1880   RICHARD ULRICH (1849–1915), an assistant in the Strasbourg Eye Clinic, began the study of aqueous humor dynamics by the use of dye injections. He used fluorescein injected subcutaneously to study normal aqueous dynamics, glaucoma, papilledema, as well as the permeability of the cornea and the lens capsule.

1880   ADOLPH ALT (1851–1920) of St. Louis published an atlas entitled *Lectures on the Human Eye in its Normal and Pathological Conditions.* This presents extensive information on ocular histology and pathology based largely on Alt's own research and experience.

1880   SIR WILLIAM BOWMAN and EDWARD NETTLESHIP (1845–1913), both surgeons to Moorfields, established the Ophthalmological Society of the United Kingdom of Great Britain. Bowman was appointed the first president.

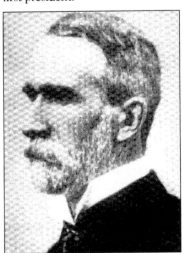

Edward Nettleship
(1845–1913)

1880   H. N. DRANSART gave the first description of frontalis suspension, using absorbable subcutaneous sutures to attach the ptotic eyelid to the brow.

1880   THOMAS R. POOLEY (1841–1926) of Brooklyn recorded his use of the sideroscope, an electromagnetic instrument that detects iron particles, to locate foreign bodies in eyes.

1881   HENRY DRURY NOYES of New York, professor of ophthalmology at the Bellevue Hospital Medical College, published his widely used and respected *A treatise on the diseases of the eye.*

1881   MARC DUFOUR (1843–1910), professor of ophthalmology at Lausanne, published *Beiträge zur Ophthalmologie* as a tribute to his teacher Friedrich Horner. Dufour also served as director of the Asile des Aveugles.

1881   ERNST FUCHS (1851–1930), professor of ophthalmology at Liège, published *Das Sarcom des Uvealtractus.* Fuchs viewed enucleation as the only treatment for uveal melanoma, and his teaching remained essentially unchallenged for nearly a century. Fuchs is considered the most influential ophthalmologist of the late nineteenth and early twentieth centuries.

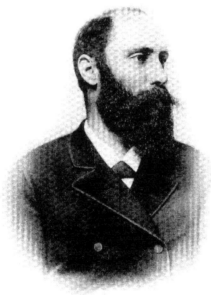

Ernst Fuchs
(1851–1930)

1881   JOSEPH LE CONTE (1823–1901), physician, physiologist, and geologist and first president of the University of California, published *Sight: an exposition of the principles of monocular and binocular vision.* He discussed the phenomena of binocular vision. The chapters on the laws of parallel and convergent motion of the eyes and the horopter are considered classics of their kind.

1881   LORD RAYLEIGH, while studying color blindness, described a number of individuals who had diminished color vision but could indistinctly see all colors. Von Kries later termed this condition 'anomalous trichromates.'

1881 WILHELM GOLDZIEHER (1849–1916) of Budapest published *Die Therpie der Augenkrankheiten*, the first Hungarian textbook of ophthalmology since Fabini's *Doctrina* (1823). The book focuses on remedies for the various diseases of the eye and includes specific prescriptions.

1882 JOHN REISBERG WOLFE published *On diseases and injuries of the eye*, intended for medical students whose specialty lay outside ophthalmology.

1882 WARREN TAY (1843–1927) at Moorfields noted a child with a peculiar white-appearing fundus and a 'cherry red spot in the fundus.' The child developed optic atrophy in four months and died 20 months later. This condition is now known as Tay–Sachs disease.

1882 A. PLACIDO of Porto, Portugal invented the keratoscope (*astigmatoscopio explorador*).

1882 DAVID HARROWER (1857–1937), a Harvard medical student studying at the Moorfields Eye Hospital, in collaboration with MR. W. JENNINGS MILLES, curator at the hospital, used the celloidin technique for fixation of the eye in the eye pathology laboratory.

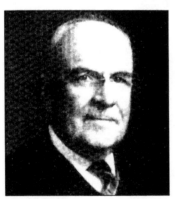

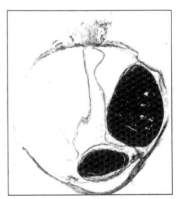

David Harrower
(1857–1937)

Cross-section of a globe from the Harrower collection

1882 THEODOR LEBER, then in Göttingen, postulated that retinal tears were due to isolated unrecognizable vitreoretinal adhesions.

1882 The *Optical Review* began as a section for opticians in a jeweler's periodical.

1882 FRIEDRICH DANIEL VON RECKLINGHAUSEN (1833–1910) in Berlin, a pupil of Virchow, gave his classic description of neurofibromatosis.

1883	ROBERT KOCH (1843–1910) of Berlin, the great pioneer in the study of infectious disease, advanced ophthalmic bacteriology with the discovery of the bacilli of two different forms of Egyptian conjunctivitis.
1883	HERMANN LUDWIG COHN (1838–1906) published *Die Hygiene des Auges in den Schulen*. The focus of the work was statistics on the rate of myopia and the consequences of print types, handwriting, eyeglasses, lighting, and seating arrangements. Cohn was a proponent of schoolchildren having regular eye examinations and developed several test-types to achieve this end. Cohn's work was influential in promoting routine eye examinations of schoolchildren in Europe and the United States.
1883	OSCAR EVERSBUSCH (1853–1912) improved Sir William Bowman's method of levator resection for the correction of ptosis, recommending advancement and folding the levator muscle by a cutaneous approach.
1883	HERMANN KUHNT (1850–1925) of Heidelberg improved on Sir William Adams's 1812 tarsal wedge resection for correction of ectropion. Kuhnt split the lid at the gray line and removed only the posterior lamella of tarsus.
1883	JULIUS VON MICHEL (1843–1911), professor of ophthalmology at Würzburg, found the tubercle bacillus, which had been discovered the previous year by Robert Koch, in enucleated eyes. This marked the beginning of Michel's extensive research on tuberculosis as a cause of uveitis.
1883	OTTO BECKER of Heidelberg published *Zu Anatomie der Gesunden und Kranken Linse*, in which he gave the name 'Morgagnian cataract' to the cataract first discovered by St. Yves in 1722. He provided a detailed description of this cataract.
1883	HENRI PARINAUD of Paris was the first to describe paralysis of convergence.
1884	MAX BURCHARDT of Berlin reported favorable results in his treatment of gonorrheal conjunctivitis by irrigation with 10% silver nitrate solution.
1884	KARL SIEGMUND FRANZ CREDÉ (1810–1892) of Berlin began instilling 2% silver nitrate solution into the eyes of newborns to prevent gonococcal infection.
1884	ALPHONSE DUBREUIL (1835–1901), surgery professor at Montpellier and a respected ophthalmic surgeon, described a procedure for simple extraction of the cataract in which he had 14 successes among 16 operations. He declared, however, that he still preferred couching and

that he had greater success with this operation.

1884   SIR HENRY ROSBOROUGH SWANZY (1844–1913) of Dublin published *A handbook of the diseases of the eye and their treatment.* This was one of the most popular English ophthalmologic textbooks of its time.

1884   ALFRED KARL VON GRAEFE (1830–1899) of Halle was among the first to introduce the principles of asepsis and antisepsis into ophthalmology.

1884   PAUL JULIUS MÖBIUS (1853–1907), a neurologist in Leipzig, gave the first description of ophthalmoplegic migraine (Möbius's disease).

1884   GEORGE LINDSAY JOHNSON (1853–1943) of Moorfields published *A new method of treating chronic glaucoma based on recent researches into its pathology.* This illustrated the increasing importance of ophthalmic pathology in shaping clinical practice.

1884   JOHN GREEN of St. Louis, apparently unaware of Streitfeild's 1872 report, described and advocated ablation of the socket.

1884   ROBERT BRUDENELL CARTER of London gave three prestigious Lettsomian lectures on 'The modern operations for cataract.' Carter advocated early surgical intervention and the use of preliminary iridectomy

1884   KARL KOLLER (1857–1944) of Vienna introduced the use of cocaine as a local anesthetic. It soon replaced ether and chloroform as the anesthetic of choice in eye surgery.

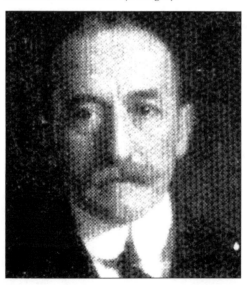

Karl Koller (1857–1944)
Courtesy of Francis A. Countway
Library of Medicine, Boston, MA

1884   ADOLPH ALT of St. Louis founded the *American Journal of*

Ophthalmology, of which he was the editor and a major contributor until 1910.

1884   JANNIK PETERSON BJERRUM (1851–1920) of Copenhagen showed that visual acuity in strabismic amblyopia is either unaffected or improved by reduced illumination.

1885   CARL FRIEDRICH OTTO WESTPHAL (1833–1890) of Berlin and LUDWIG EDINGER (1855–1918) of Frankfurt independently provided much of the early information on the neuronal mass that forms the oculomotor nucleus (Edinger–Westphal nucleus).

1885   ERNST FUCHS published his monograph entitled *The causes and prevention of blindness*. This study, based on his own clinical experience and a review of the literature, gained Fuchs wide recognition and a prize of 80 francs offered by the Society for the Prevention of Blindness in London.

1885   DR. MYLES STANDISH, an ophthalmology intern at the Massachusetts Eye and Ear Infirmary, was excited by an article written by W. JENNINGS MILLES in the *British Medical Journal* regarding the use of celloidin for embedding ocular tissue. Standish wrote to Milles and received the necessary information and subsequently was the first pathologist in America to use celloidin for embedding ocular specimens.

1885   EDWARD JACKSON (1856–1942) of Philadelphia devised a method of retinoscopy (skiascopy) using a plane mirror rather than the concave mirror, which was applicable to all forms of ametropia.

1885   JULIUS HIRSCHBERG, professor at the University of Berlin, introduced the electromagnet into ophthalmology with his publication *Der Electromagnet in der Augenheilkunde*.

1885   W. S. DENNETT (d. 1925) of New York City demonstrated the first electric ophthalmoscope to the American Ophthalmologic Society. The instrument was attached by wires to a battery and used a bulb with a short-lived filament. Due to the inadequacies of the lamp and the size and heavy weight of the battery, his invention was not enthusiastically received.

1885   WILLIAM STUART HALSTEAD (1852–1992), professor of surgery at Johns Hopkins University, developed nerve-blocking conduction anesthesia after hazardous experimentation on himself. CRILE (1897) and CUSHING (1900) put conduction anesthesia into general practice.

1885   PHILIP HENRY MULES (1843–1905) of Manchester devised an early evisceration operation with insertion of a hollow glass sphere into the scleral sac.

1885 Jakob Stilling, professor of ophthalmology in Strasbourg, cited the anatomical configuration of the orbits to be the cause of concomitant squint.

1885 Sir Jonathan Hutchinson in London theorized that sympathetic ophthalmitis was caused by 'infective cells' from the diseased eye selectively spreading to the healthy eye through the bloodstream in a process distinct from bacterial septicemia.

1885 Robert Walter Doyne (1857–1916), after working as a surgeon in the Royal Navy, established an eye clinic that became the Oxford Eye Hospital.

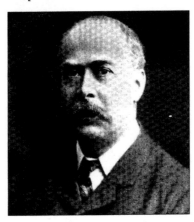

Robert Walter Doyne
(1857–1916)

1885 William Adams Frost (1853–1935), at Moorfields, proposed placing a hollow glass ball in Tenon's capsule following enucleation. Frost sutured the horizontal and vertical recti over the implant.

1886 Jannik Peterson Bjerrum of Copenhagen began his study of visual field defects in glaucoma by quantitative perimetry on a tangent screen and discovered the 'Bjerrum scotoma.'

1886 Paul Haensell (1840–1912), an ophthalmologist and histologist in Paris, wrote a series of papers describing a microtome for cutting eye sections, methods of embedding the eye in paraffin and celloidin, and the preservation of eye specimens. In addition, he was the first to apply the recently invented rotary microtome to the study of the eye.

1886 At the Heidelberg Ophthalmic Society meeting, Arthur von Hippel of Königsberg exhibited a young girl in whom he transplanted a full-thickness rabbit cornea into a lamellar bed. The patient's vision was improved from counting fingers at 2 meters to 20/200.

1886 Hermann Schmidt-Rimpler, director of the eye clinic at the University of Marburg, published *Augenheilkunde und Ophthalmoskopie* that stressed the increasingly recognized relationship between eye diseases and general organic disease.

1886   PHOTINOS PANAS proposed a frontalis muscle (brow) suspension operation involving burying deepithelialized skin strips raised from the lid crease and attached to the brow by tunneling subcutaneously. This transposition of biological material to transmit the force of the frontalis to the eyelid constituted a major conceptual advance in the correction of ptosis.

1886   JOHN ELMER WEEKS (1853–1949) of New York City isolated the bacterium responsible for acute epidemic conjunctivitis, *Haemophilus aegyptius*, or Koch–Weeks bacillus, and transmitted the disease to volunteers, including himself. To isolate the organism, Weeks developed new laboratory culture techniques that contributed to microbiology in general.

1886   CARL WEDL and EMIL BOCK (1857–1916), at the University of Vienna, published an atlas entitled *Atlas zur pathologischen Anatomie des Auges*. The book was overshadowed by Pagenstecher and Genth's 1875 atlas and received little attention.

1886   HERMANN VON HELMHOLTZ was awarded the Graefe Medal at the Heidelberg Ophthalmological Society for the invention of the ophthalmoscope. Frans Cornelis Donders declared Helmholtz had 'unfolded to us a new world!'

1886   JOHN HUGHLINGS JACKSON presented the Bowman lecture on 'Ophthalmology and diseases of the nervous system.' Jackson concluded that the cerebral cortex played a significant role in a number of visual activities but did not believe in clearly delineated autonomous information centers.

1886   OTTO HAAB (1850–1931), professor of ophthalmology at the University of Zurich, described the phenomenon now known as Habb's reflex.

1886   GILES CHRISTOPHER SAVAGE (1854–1930) was appointed professor of ophthalmology at Vanderbilt University. Savage, born in Mississippi, was representative of the better-trained American ophthalmologists of his day. He studied first at Jefferson Medical College and then in London and Vienna.

1887   SWAN MOSES BURNETT (1847–1906), a native Tennessee ophthalmologist, published *A theoretical and practical treatise on astigmatism*. It discussed the causes, examination, and diagnosis of astigmatism, which he characterized as 'paradoxical manifestations.' Burnett also studied refraction and the statistical frequency of ocular diseases between races.

1887	RUDOLF BERLIN in Stuttgart published *Eine besondere Art der Wortblindheit (Dyslexie)*. This introduced the term 'dyslexia,' which Berlin describes in this work as a disease of the brain.
1887	OTTO LANGE (1852–1913), an ophthalmologist in Braunschweig, published *Topographische Anatomie des menschlichen Orbitalinhalts*. In the same year, he helped establish a journal entitled *Mittheilungen aus der St. Petersburger Augen-Heilanstalt*. He contributed the article 'Über Glaukom.'
1887	THEODORE DUNHAM of New York suggested the use of a vascularized pedicle flap for eye reconstruction.
1887	ÉMIL BERGER (1855–1926) published *Beiträge zur Anatomie des Agues in normalen und pathologischem Zustande*. This work focused on the pathology of eye disease.
1887	EDWARD TREACHER COLLINS (1862–1937) was appointed as pathologist and curator of the museum at Moorfields. His work with both gross specimens and microscopic examination drew wide recognition and formed the basis for his important text *Researches into the anatomy and pathology of the eye* (1896).
1887	F. E. MÜLLER, an artificial eye maker in Wiesbaden, devised the first contact lens at the request of THEODOR SAEMISCH. The lens, made of glass, was used not to correct vision but to protect the cornea of a patient with no eyelids.
1887	The New York Medical Society, under the leadership of LUCIEN HOWE (1848–1928), formed a working group to study blindness resulting from ophthalmia neonatorum. This led to legislation throughout the United States requiring silver nitrate prophylaxis.
1887	ERNEST MOTAIS (1845–1913), professor of ophthalmology in Angiers, France, published *L'anatomie de l'apparat moteur de l'oeil de l'homme et des vertébrés*, an outstanding discussion of the anatomy and physiology of the extraocular muscles that included his own original observations.
1887	ROBERT BRUDENELL CARTER and WILLIAM ADAMS FROST, both at St. George's Hospital in London, published *Ophthalmic surgery*.
1887	EDWARD NETTLESHIP, a surgeon at Moorfields, published the first description of diabetic microaneurysms.
1887	LUCIEN HOWE of Buffalo succeeded in photographing the human fundus oculi.
1887	WILLIAM LANG (1863–1937) devised the Frost–Lang method of orbital implants after enucleation, following Frost's method of placing a glass ball within Tenon's capsule by modifying it to include suturing

Edward Treacher Collins
(1862–1937)

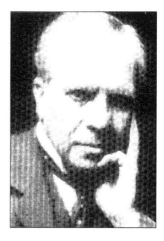

Lucien Howe
(1848–1928)

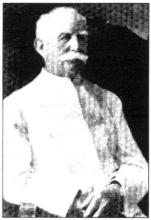

Ernest Motais
(1845–1913)

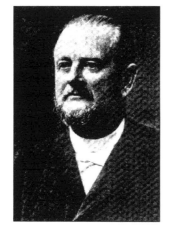

Tenon's capsule as well.

1887	GEORGE THOMAS STEVENS (1832–1921) of New York published *Functional diseases of the nervous system* that emphasized the causal role that strabismus and refractive errors play in neurological disorders such as epilepsy and chorea.
1887	BERNHARD SACHS (b. 1858) described amaurotic family idiocy (Tay–Sachs disease), the ocular manifestations of which had been noted in 1880 by WARREN TAY.
1887	CARL FRIEDRICH OTTO WESTPHAL, professor of psychiatry in Berlin, first reported of the identification of a nucleus for pupillary constriction in the adult brain.
1888	The American Medical Association Section on Ophthalmology, Otolaryngology, and Laryngology was divided into two sections: one known as Ophthalmology and the other as Laryngology and Otology.
1888	ARTHUR VON HIPPEL of Giessen reported two successful keratoplasties in humans in which the graft remained clear and there was functional visual improvement. Hippel devised a circular trephine that became the prototype for modern trephines.
1888	ADOLF VOSSIUS (1855–1925), professor of ophthalmology at the Universities of Königsburg, published *Grundriss der Augenheilkunde*. Vossius gave the earliest report of annular contusion cataract, i.e. Vossius's lenticular ring, and keratitis interstitialis centralis annularis.
1888	GEORGE MILBRY GOULD (1848–1922) received his medical degree from Jefferson Medical College and began his ophthalmology practice in Philadelphia. He wrote on a number of ophthalmology subjects and drew many adherents to his belief that errors of refraction negatively affect general health. In a four-volume series, Gould ascribed the morbid psychology and neurotic symptoms of certain well-known persons to the effects of asthenopia dependent upon astigmatism and other errors of refraction.
1888	RUDOLF ULRICH KRÖNLEIN (1847–1910) in Germany developed lateral orbitotomy surgery to take out orbital dermoid cysts. His incisional technique was modified by Emil Theodor Kocher in Bern and more recently by Raymond Berke to reduce scarring and increase orbital access.
1888	MAX KNIES in Freiberg published *Grundriss der Augenheilkunde*, an important work in establishing the relationship of diseases of the eye to systemic diseases. A second part was published in 1893.
1888	AUGUST WAGENMANN (1862–1955) carried out experiments in rabbits that demonstrated that a portion of the cornea excised in its

entire thickness, when reinserted, could heal in place and remain transparent. Wagenmann recognized that, contrary to Hippel's claim, the gap in Descemet's membrane was bridged by newly formed endothelium.

1888   ADOLF EUGEN FICK (1852–1937) of Zurich published a paper describing his use of glass lenses covering the cornea to correct irregular astigmatism. ERNST ABBE, the director of the Zeiss Optical factories at Jena, supplied the lenses. Fick coined the term 'contact lens.'

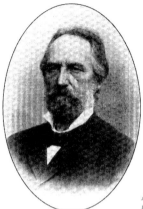

Adolf Eugen Fick
(1852–1937)

1888   *The Collected Papers of Sir W. Bowman, Bart., F.R.S.* was issued by an international committee seeking to honor the 72-year-old giant in ophthalmology. The two volumes cover, among other subjects, color blindness, glaucoma iridectomy, epiphora, and artificial pupils.

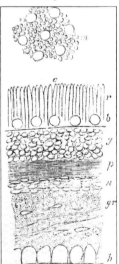

Illustration of Jacob's Membrane from *The Collected Papers of Sir W. Bowman, Bart., F.R.S.* (1888) by Sir William Bowman

| 1888 | JEAN BAPTISTE EUGENE KALT (1861–1941) of Paris was one of the first to use contact lenses in the treatment of keratoconus. |

| 1889 | HENRI PARINAUD in Paris described an infectious conjunctivitis transmitted to the human eye from animals. This conjuctivitis is associated with swelling of the preauricular and submandibular lymph nodes. |

| 1889 | JOSEPH PRIESTLEY SMITH of Birmingham, in his Erasmus Wilson lectures delivered before the Royal College of Surgeons, theorized that as one gets older the circumlental space narrows and results in a predilection toward glaucoma. |

| 1889 | LEOPOLD KÖNIGSTEIN (1850–1924), a lecturer in ophthalmology at the University of Vienna, published the first volume of his *Die Behandlung der häufigsten und wichtigsten Augenkrankheiten*. Königstein focuses on anatomical and physiological as well as clinical aspects of ophthalmology and includes his original observations on the physiology and pathology of the lens. |

| 1889 | GEORGE THOMAS STEVENS of New York City joined a trial study with a committee, composed of members of the New York Neurological Society, assigned to assess the effectiveness of his methods of treating neurological disorders by attention to phorias and refractive errors. After two and a half years, the study was ended as the committee decided that the treatment did not adequately alleviate the symptoms. |

| 1889 | JANNIK PETERSON BJERRUM of Copenhagen published 'An addition to the usual examination of the visual field and the visual field in glaucoma' in the *Nordisk Ophthalmologisk Tidskrift*. His paper analyzed visual field defects using quantitative perimetry. His technique was widely used for the following 40 years and has been continually used since then. |

| 1889 | CHARLES HORACE MAYO (1865–1959), surgeon and cofounder of the Mayo Clinic, operated on his first ophthalmic patient at St. Mary's Hospital in Rochester. The enucleation of the eye was successful, and his father and brother determined that Charles should take charge of all ocular procedures. |

| 1889 | ERNEST EDMUND MADDOX (1860–1933), ophthalmic surgeon to the Royal Edinburgh Infirmary, published his innovative teachings on the diagnosis and treatment of anomalies of the extrinsic muscles of the eye in his textbook *The clinical use of prisms and the decentering of lenses*. Maddox introduced a method of photographing the corneal reflexes in squint. |

| 1889 | LOUIS DE WECKER of Paris published *Manuel d'Ophthalmologie* in which he described an instrument for examining the cornea. It |

consisted of a tube with an eyepiece, an objective, and an adjustable condensing lens from which light was reflected.

1889   ERNST FUCHS, professor in Vienna, published the first edition of his *Lehrbuch der Augenheilkunde*, an extremely influential text.

1889   FREDERICK HERMANN VERHOEFF (1874–1968) from Louisville, Kentucky graduated from the new Johns Hopkins Medical School and accepted a position as assistant surgeon at the Baltimore Eye, Ear, and Throat Charity Hospital. He was the first Hopkins medical graduate to enter ophthalmology.

1889   ALLVAR GULLSTRAND (1862–1930) at Uppsala, Sweden designed an ophthalmometric apparatus for calculating corneal astigmatism.

1889   HEINRICH LEOPOLD SCHÖLER (1844–1918), professor of ophthalmology in Berlin, in his *Zur operativen Behandlung und Heilung der Netzhautablösung* suggested, in treating retinal detatchment, the injection of a few drops of iodine into the preretinal space to eliminate vitreous traction and to cause an adhesion between the retina and choroids.

1889   SIR JONATHAN HUTCHINSON began publication of *Archives of Surgery* in ten volumes. This became a compendium of Hutchinson's original observations, many of which concerned ophthalmology.

1890   ADOLF BECK (1863–1942), a Polish neurophysiologist, confirmed and expanded on Caton's work showing electrical differences in the posterior cortex following visual stimulation.

1890   ERNEST EDMUND MADDOX invented the 'double prism Maddox rod' for ocular motility testing.

1890   SIR JONATHAN HUTCHINSON of London reported the first case of temporal arteritis in the *Archives of Surgery* but attributed the cause to wearing a too-tight hat.

1890   CHARLES F. PRENTICE (1854–1946), a New York engineer and optician, published 'A metric system of numbering and measuring prisms,' in which he introduced his famous Prentice's Rule of decentration.

1890   HENRY DRURY NOYES of New York published his *Text-book on diseases of the eye*, a much expanded and updated revision of his 1881 *Treatise*.

1890   XAVIER GALEZOWSKI of Paris attempted retinal suturing to affix the detached retina to the eye wall. His catgut suture went through the sclera, retina, and vitreous cavity and exited through the sclera.

1890   Intracapsular cataract extraction regained favor as the British Indian Medical Service reported their successes. Its most prominent advocate was COLONEL HENRY SMITH (1857–1948), who practiced in the Punjab. He expressed the lens in its capsule by pressure.

1891   AMY STOKES BARTON (1841–1900), the first woman to practice ophthalmology in Pennsylvania, was appointed clinical professor of ophthalmology at Women's Medical College of Pennsylvania.

1891   JOSEPH PRIESTLEY SMITH of Birmingham published *On the pathology and treatment of glaucoma*. Smith was the inventor of the modern perimeter and a popular tonometer.

1891   FREDERICK WILLIAM EDRIDGE-GREEN (1863–1953), medical officer at the Northumberland House Asylum, published *Colour-blindness and colour-perception*. This introduced his color vision lantern test, which was officially adopted in Great Britain in 1945 in place of the Homgren vision lantern test.

1891   ERIK JOHAN WIDMARK (1850–1909), professor of ophthalmic and general surgery at the Karolinska Medical-Surgical Institute in Sweden, published *Beiträge zur Ophthalmologie*. Widmark studied snow blindness, ultraviolet radiation, 'ophthalmia electrica,' and the pathogenic effects of ultraviolet radiation on the eyes and skin.

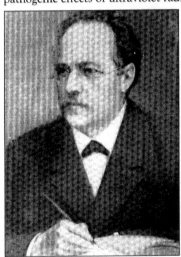

Erik Johan Widmark
(1850–1909)

1891   ANATOLE PIERRE LOUIS GILLET DE GRANDMONT (1837–1894) of Paris illustrated his partial resection of the upper tarsus and resection of Müller's muscle for the treatment of ptosis.

1891   FERDINAND SUAREX DE MENDOZA recommended for the first time preplacing the limbal sutures in a cataract operation.

1891   OTTO HAAB, professor of ophthalmology at the University of Zurich, described Galvanic cautery as a method of temporarily closing canaliculi before intraocular surgery for patients with dacryocystitis. He achieved permanent closure of the canaliculi by inserting the cautery tip approximately 5 mm into the canal, a procedure still used today for patients with dry eye syndrome.

1891   The journal *Ophthalmic Record* was established and continued publication until 1918. Its first editor was GILES CHRISTOPHER SAVAGE, professor of ophthalmology at Vanderbilt University.

1891   HENRI PARINAUD of Paris concluded that concomitant squint was due to a deficiency or disturbance of the central nervous system rather than a defect in the muscles themselves.

1891   *The Optician*, a journal devoted to optics and vision, began publication.

1892   HUGO FRIEDRICH MAGNUS (1842–1907) of Germany, professor of ophthalmology in Breslau, published the initial section of his 20-part collaborative work *Augenärztliche unterrichtstafeln für den akademischen und selbst-unterricht*. Other contributors were KARL BAAS, WILHELM CZERMAK, CARL RICHARD GREEFF, OTTO HAAG, EDMUND LANDOLT, MAXIMILLIAN SALZMANN, and ADOLF VOSSIUS. The final sections appeared in 1900.

1892   OTTO HAAB of Zurich designed a powerful magnet for extracting foreign bodies from the eye.

1892   GEORGE EDMUND DE SCHWEINITZ (1858–1938) authored *Diseases of the Eye*, which for the next three decades was considered one of the most authoritative American works in the field.

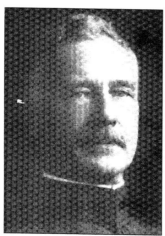

George Edmund de Schweinitz
(1858–1938)

1892   The journal *Annals of Ophthalmology* was established by JAMES P. PARKER of St. Louis.

1892   JOSEF BAYER (1847–1925) of Vienna, trained in both human and veterinary medicine, issued *Bildiche Darstellung des gesunden und kranken Auges unserer Hausthiere*, a major eye pathology work on animals that was considered the veterinary counterpart of Wedl and Bock's 1886 atlas. Bayer assembled a notable museum to house his collection of diseased eyes enucleated from animals.

1892   FÉLIX LAGRANGE (1855–1928), professor of surgery at the University of Bordeaux, published his important text on tumors of the eye and orbit, *Études sur les tumeurs de l'oeil, de l'orbite et des annexes.*

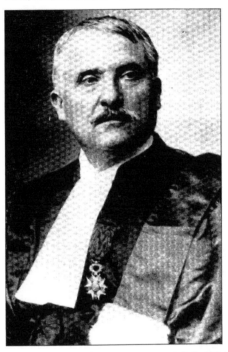

Félix Lagrange
(1855–1928)

1892   EDWARD TREACHER COLLINS and F. R. CROSS described two cases of epithelial implantation in the anterior chamber following cataract.

1893   SIEGFRIED CZAPSKI (1861–1907), a German instrument maker and researcher, published *Theorie der optischen Instrumente nach Abbe*, which presents the principles of optics and of optical instruments. He describes prisms, lenses, microscopes, and magnifying glasses.

1893   A collected edition of key works leading to the development of the ophthalmoscope by WILLIAM CUMMING, HERMANN VON HELMHOLTZ, CHRISTIAN GEORGE THEODORE RUETE, and ERNST WILHELM VON BRÜCKE was published as *Das Augenleuchten und die Erfindung des Augenspiegels dargestellt in Abhandlungen.*

| 1893 | WILHELM WUNDT (1832–1920) of Leipzig proposed a photochemical explanation of color perception that held that retinal excitation occurs through a chromatic and an achromatic stimulation brought about by photochemical reaction within the retinal elements. |

1893   WILHELM WUNDT (1832–1920) of Leipzig proposed a photochemical explanation of color perception that held that retinal excitation occurs through a chromatic and an achromatic stimulation brought about by photochemical reaction within the retinal elements.

1893   GASPARINE isolated the pneumococcus as a causative factor in various types of corneal ulcers.

1893   GILES CHRISTOPHER SAVAGE, professor of ophthalmology at Vanderbilt University, published *New Truths in Ophthalmology*, which discussed the 'functions of the oblique muscles' and other issues in 'ophthalmic myology.' He studied also the heterophorias (which he named) and the role of ocular motility in eyestrain.

1893   J. BLUM and his son FERDINAND BLUM (1865–1959), physicians in Frankfurt, introduced formaldehyde fixation into histopathology.

1893   GEORGE H. MONKS of Boston first described the use of an arterialized pedicle flap from the scalp to reconstruct the lower lid.

1893   JEAN BAPTISTE EUGENE KALT described blown glass contact lenses for improvement of vision for patients with keratoconus. In contrast to Fick's lenses, which had a scleral flange, Kalt's lenses covered only the cornea.

1893   GUILLOT in Nancy produced what contemporaries claimed were the first 'usable' photos of the human ocular fundus six years after Lucian Howe's success. Guillot used a mirror reflex camera and magnesium powder that produced a flash synchronously with the mirror being flipped out of the way.

1893   According to Schepens, ALIMO described a technique of full-thickness scleral resection for the treatment of retinal detachments.

1893   CARL VON HESS (1863–1923) of Munich described a surgical treatment of ptosis in which the lid was attached to the brow by a subcutaneous suture, which was removed after several weeks. This was a modification of an earlier procedure reported by H. N. Dransart in 1880 in which the lid was attached to the brow by an absorbable subcutaneous suture. Both techniques depended on the formation of sufficient scar tissue along the suture tracks to elevate the lid permanently.

1893   GEORGES GAZÉPY (1860–1929) published his papers on alcohol–tobacco amblyopia, hysterical amblyopia, hemeralopia, and congenital eye diseases in the *Annales d'Oculistique*.

1894   GEORGE EDMUND DE SCHWEINITZ, professor of ophthalmology at the Philadelphia Polyclinic, received the Alvarenga Prize from the College of Physicians of Philadelphia for his important monograph

Toxic amblyopias. This treatise included de Schweinitz's original research on quinine-induced amblyopia in dogs.

1894   ADOLF EUGEN FICK published his influential *Lehrbuch der Augenheilkunde.* The book was notable for its sections on objective methods of examination and function tests.

1894   SANTIAGO RAMÓN Y CAJAL (1852–1934) of Spain, neurohistologist, published his classic account of the structure of the vertebrate retina.

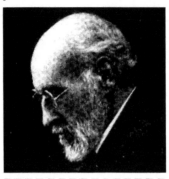

Santiago Ramón y Cajal
(1852–1934)

1894   PHOTINOS PANAS, professor of ophthalmology at the University of Paris, published *Traité des maladies des yeux,* the best French textbook of ophthalmology to appear during this period.

1894   KONRAD ZENKER described a tissue fixative for histopathology containing potassium bichromate and bichloride of mercury, now known as Zenker's solution.

1894   JEAN BAPTISTE EUGÈNE KALT of Paris reintroduced Henry Willard Williams's cataract wound sutures, employing corneoscleral sutures.

1894   CARL LUDWIG SCHLIECH in Germany described infiltration anesthesia with cocaine.

1894   FRIEDRICH DIMMER (1855–1926) of Vienna advanced knowledge of

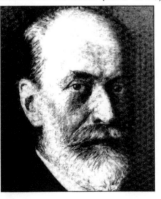

Friedrich Dimmer
(1855–1926)

the anatomy and physiology of the macula with his detailed study *Beitrage zur Anatomie und Physiologie der Macula lutea des Menschen.*

1894   CASEY ALBERT WOOD (1856–1942) of Chicago published his findings on the effects of methyl alcohol on the optic nerve in *The toxic amblyopias.*

1895   EUGEN VON HIPPEL (1867–1939), a student of Leber at Heidelberg, gave the first description of angiomatosis retinae (Hippel's disease).

1895   OTTO HAAB of Zurich published *Atlas of ophthalmology* in German and English editions. This book described the methods of conducting an ophthalmoscopic examination and the appearance of the normal and diseased fundus. This was the first of Haab's popular series of atlases covering external diseases, surgery of the eye, and other aspects of ophthalmology.

1895   BERNHARD SACHS published the earliest American treatise on the nervous diseases of children. The was based on his ophthalmic practice during the years of 1887–1895 and included reports of 'amaurotic family idiocy' (Tay–Sachs disease).

1895   EDWARD JACKSON of Philadelphia published *Skiascopy and its practical application to the study of refraction,* an important book that detailed his technique using the reflex from a plane mirror to determine the refractive error.

1895   The *Optical Journal,* a periodical devoted to optics and vision, begins to appear.

1895   WILHELM KONRAD RÖNTGEN, professor of physics at Würzburg, while experimenting with a Crookes tube, produced a new kind of ray which he called X-rays (Röntgen rays).

1896   JOHANN NEPOMUK OELLER (1850–1932), a lecturer on ophthalmology in München, began publication of his *Atlas der Ophthalmoscopie.* The plates were lithographed after Oeller's own oil sketches and provide greater detail and more intense color than previous fundus atlases. The last of the fourteen parts (74 plates) was issued in 1924.

1896   VINCENZ FUKALA (1847–1911), an ophthalmologist in Vienna, published *Heilung höchstgradiger Kurzsichtigkeit,* which describes 'Fukala's operation' for myopia. This consists of discission and extraction of the lens for relief of severe myopia.

1896   ADOLF WEBER of Darmstadt introduced the use of pilocarpine, a jaborandi plant extract, for glaucoma therapy.

1896   HARDY and GERARD introduced pilocarpine to general medicine. This drug was derived from the leaves and bark of a South American plant of the rue family, *Pilocarpus pinnatus.*

1896 ARTHUR GROENOUW (1862–1945) of Breslau published *Anleitung zur Berechnung der Erwerbsfähigkeitbei Sehstörungen*, which included his studies on the toxic amblyopias.

1896 VICTOR MORAX (1866–1935), at the Institute Pasteur in Paris, isolated a diplobacillus causing chronic conjunctivitis, *Moraxella lacunata*. THEODOR AXENFELD (1867–1930) at Freiburg independently isolated this bacterium the following year.

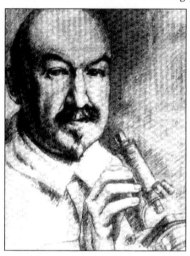

Victor Morax
(1866–1935)

1896 HUGO WOLFF in Berlin reported an aponeurosis shortening technique for the treatment of ptosis that is similar to modern procedures.

1896 JOSEPH PRIESTLEY SMITH in Birmingham supported Parinaud's conclusion (1891) that concomitant squint is due to a disturbance of the central nervous system.

1896 FELIX DE LAPERSONNE (1853–1937), professor of ophthalmology in Paris, proposed a ptosis procedure involving true levator resection and advancement by an external approach.

1896 The American Optical Company received a patent for its Axonometer, the first instrument to determine graphically the optical centers and axes of lenses.

1896 EDWARD TREACHER COLLINS, pathologist and curator of the museum at Moorfields, published *Researches into the anatomy and pathology of the eye*. This work is considered the first 'modern' single-volume text on the histopathology of the eye.

1896 WILLIAM ADAMS FROST of Moorfields published *The fundus oculi, with an ophthalmoscopic atlas*. Until the electric ophthalmoscope provided finer details, the plates in this work, reproduced by color lithography after the drawings of A.W. HEAD, provided the finest illustrations of the fundus.

1896   DANIEL VAN DUYSE (1852–1924) of Ghent used the new invention of the X-ray to produce the first radiograph that showed a foreign body in an eye. In the same year, he founded the Belgium Ophthalmological Society.

1896   CHARLES HERBERT WILLIAMS (1850–1918) of Boston, using a Crookes tube to generate X-rays, obtained an image of an intraocular foreign body in a 17-year-old boy.

1896   THEODOR LEBER, professor of ophthalmology at Heidelberg, was awarded the second Graefe medal for his contributions on disorders of the ocular circulation, the degeneration of retinal pigment, color vision in diseases of the retina, pathologic changes in the ocular fluids, and the diabetic disorders of the eye.

1896   ROBERT WALTER DOYNE, senior surgeon at the Oxford Eye Hospital, published *Notes on the more common diseases of the eye*, a concise discussion of the diagnosis and treatment of commonly encountered eye problems intended for the general physician.

1896   CHARLES F. PRENTICE, an engineer and optician, and ANDREW JAY CROSS, who practiced optometry in California, lobbied for regulatory legislation for optometry in the state of New York, but no bill was passed until 1908.

1896   American ophthalmologists hosted the Fifth International Congress of Ophthalmology in New York.

1896   The Western Ophthalmological, Otological, Laryngological, and Rhinological Association, precursor to the American Academy of Ophthalmology and Otolaryngology, was organized by HAL FORESTER in Kansas City. Meeting papers and proceedings were published in the *American Journal of Ophthalmology* and the *Laryngoscope*.

1897   E. BOECKMANN published an article in the *Journal of the American Medical Association* that detailed his pterygia surgery technique. This was one of the first descriptions of pterygia treatments in English literature.

1897–1900   WILLIAM FISHER NORRIS and CHARLES A. OLIVER (1853–1911) coedited *A system of diseases of the eye*. This contained chapters from international leaders in ophthalmology. The set was considered an American counterpart to Graefe-Saemisch's *Handbuch der Gesamten Augenheilkunde*.

1897   EDMOND LANDOLT (1846–1926) of Paris, in his *Therapeutisches*

Taschenbuch für Augenärzte, concurs with Stilling's theory that concomitant squint is the result of the anatomical configuration of the orbits.

1897   ERNEST MOTAIS of Angiers, France and HENRI PARINAUD of Paris independently proposed a new form of ptosis repair by suspending the lid from the superior rectus muscle. This technique proved capable of providing good cosmetic results, but the blink was hampered and lid closure was incomplete.

1897   WILLIAM MERRICK SWEET (1860–1926) of Philadelphia devised a method for localizing foreign bodies in the eye by means of X-rays that was the standard for many years.

1897   SIEGFRIED CZAPSKI, a German instrument maker and researcher, invented a corneal microscope in which binocular vision was obtained by using a combination of two microscopes and the illumination of an electric lamp.

1897   SIR CHARLES SCOTT SHERRINGTON (1857–1952), a physiology professor at Liverpool and Oxford, published his landmark paper on reciprocal innervation of antagonistic muscles, establishing the concept that when one set of muscles is stimulated the opposing set is inhibited in reflex.

1898   MARIUS HANS ERIK TSCHERNING (1854–1939), working in Paris, published *Optique physiologique dioptrique oculaire-Fonctions de la rétine-Les mouvements oculaires et la vision vinoculaire; Leçons professées a la Sorbonee*. Included are the studies using afterimages to observe torsion in oblique movements of the eye.

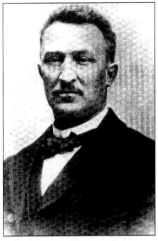

Marius Hans Erik Tscherning
(1854–1939)

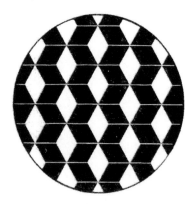

Illustration from *Optique physiologique dioptrique oculaire-Fonctions de la rétine-Les mouvements oculaires et la vision vinoculaire; Leçons professées a la Sorbonee* (1898) by Tscherning

1898	CARL RICHARD GREEFF (1862–1938) of Berlin published *Anleitung zur mikroskopischen Untersuchung des Auges*, an important contribution to the pathologic histology of the eye.
1898	ALEXIOS TRANTAS (1867–1960), an ophthalmologist in Constantinople, became the first person to observe the angle of the interior chamber while examining the eye in a living patient with a very deep chamber. He used an ophthalmoscope and facilitated the observation by applying digital pressure, which allowed for easier viewing of the angle. He published his findings in 1901 and 1907, which included extending the viewing to include the pars plana, ciliary body, and the anterior of the retina.
1898	LENDERT JAN LANS, a Dutch ophthalmologist, published 'Experimental studies of the treatment of astigmatism with non-perforating corneal incision.' This established numerous principles of astigmatic and radial keratotomy.
1898	ERNEST EDMUND MADDOX, ophthalmic surgeon to the Royal Edinburgh Infirmary, published *Tests and studies of the ocular muscles*. This was an important contribution to the objective testing of ocular motility. In the same year, he invented the Maddox tangent scale.
1898	Local organizing and lobbying for legislation allowing for the professionalization of optometry resulted in the formation of a national organization, The American Association of Opticians, which held its first meeting in New York City. Anyone interested in optics could be a member.
1898	The Western Ophthalmological, Otological, Laryngological, and Rhinological Association, now a thriving organization, renames itself the Western Ophthalmological and Otolaryngological Association. Presentations at the Western Ophthalmological and Otolaryngological Association were segregated into those on nose and throat and those on the eye and ear.
1898	Publication of the second edition of the Graefe-Saemisch *Handbuch der Gesamten Augenheilkunde* was begun but not completed owing to the death of THEODOR SAEMISCH in 1909.
1898	JOHN COUPER, a prominent ophthalmic surgeon at Moorfields, supported equality of women on the staff of that institution.
1898	DOUGLAS ARGYLL ROBERTSON of Edinburgh described a procedure for repair of lower lid ectropion. He utilized a skin strip to support the lid vertically and laterally and employed a full-thickness excision of the eyelid to correct the horizontal laxity.
1899	HERMAN WILDBRAND (1851–1935) of Breslau and ALFRED SAENGER

produced the first of their nine-volume set, *The Neurology of the Eye: A Handbook for Neurologists and Ophthalmologists.*

1899   HOWARD FORDE HANSELL (1855–1934) and WENDELL REBER of Philadelphia co-authored *A practical handbook of the muscular anomalies of the eye* that gave current information on the diagnoses and treatment of abnormal states of the eye muscles.

1899   KARL WILHELM VON ZEHENDER of Munich improved Liebreich's binocular microscope by attaching an electric light for illumination.

1899   HERMANN SCHMIDT-RIMPLER at Halle rediscovered Sichel's 'herniated orbital fat,' which he called 'Fett-hernien,' and discussed its significance and management.

1899   HAROLD GIFFORD (1858–1929) of Omaha advocated treating sympathetic ophthalmitis with large amounts of sodium salicylate. This was claimed to be effective in delaying the symptoms. Gifford believed sympathetic ophthalmia to be due to an organism that spread from the injured eye to the fellow eye.

1900   JEAN DARIER (1856–1939) of Paris discovered the hypotensive effect of sympathomimetic drugs in the course of clinical trials in which adrenal extracts were topically applied to the treatment of inflammatory diseases of the anterior segment of the eye.

1900   CHARLES HENRY MAY (1861–1943), director of ophthalmology at Bellevue, published *Manual of Diseases of the Eye*, a popular textbook for medical students.

1900   ALLVAR GULLSTRAND, professor of ophthalmology in Uppsala, published *Allgemeine Theorie der monochromatischen Aberrationen und ihre nächstein Ergebnisse für die Ophthalmologie.*

1900   JAMES P. PARKER of St. Louis and WILLIAM MERRICK SWEET of Philadelphia developed the first hand-held magnet for use in extracting foreign bodies from eyes.

1900   FRITZ SALZER (1867–1952) in Germany began publication of a series of articles spanning nearly four decades that made clear distinctions among the various types of donor material: *autoplasty, homoplasty and heteroplasty.* He stated that from a practical standpoint, the best source for a corneal graft was fresh human tissue and suggested fresh tissue be obtained from an embryo or stillborn infant.

1900   ANDRÉ MAGITOT (1877–1958) of Paris proposed his theory that aqueous humor was 'a stagnant dialysate of the plasma.' His plasma transudate theory, although it was incorrect, was supported by Leber and Starling and was championed in the 1920s and 1930s by Sir Stewart Duke-Elder (1898–1978).

1900   FRIEDRICH DIMMER, professor of ophthalmology at Graz, demonstrated his technique for photographing the ocular fundus at the International Congress of Ophthalmology at Utrecht.

1900   ALEXIOS TRANTAS in Constantinople suggested the use of scleral depression to provide a view of the fundus periphery.

1900   COLONEL HENRY SMITH of the British Indian Medical Service published a description of the 'Smith-Indian' cataract extraction technique. His method consists of making a large corneal incision, with or without an iridectomy, and the luxation of the lens by a specially devised spatula and a large strabismus hook.

1900   WILHELM GOLDZIEHER of Budapest developed a 'lid crutch,' which supplanted Auguste Bérard's lid clamp treatment for levator paralysis.

1901   JOHN HERBERT PARSONS (1868–1957) was appointed curator of the museum at Moorfields Eye Hospital. This launched Parsons's career as a superb clinical and experimental eye pathologist.

1901   RENÉ LE FORT (1869–1951) of Lille, France published his study of the lines of greatest weakness in the midface region in relation to orbital trauma.

1901   GEORGE LINDSAY JOHNSON, a surgeon at Moorfields, published 'Contributions to the comparative anatomy of the mammalian eye, chiefly based on ophthalmological examination.' Johnson spent most of his spare time at the London zoo pursuing his interest in the comparative anatomy of the eye.

1901   Minnesota became the first state to establish regulatory guidelines for optometry, followed by California and North Dakota.

1901   HUGO WOLFF of Berlin modified the hand ophthalmoscope to produce a focal beam of illumination on the retina.

1901   FRIEDRICH BEST (1871–1965) of Dresden discovered a new staining technique for glygogen that facilitated the distinction of rods and cones.

1902   STOEWER in Germany invented the phacoeresis technique for applying traction with a suction cup in intracapsular lens extraction.

1902   WILLIAM JOHN ADIE (1886–1935), an Australian on the staff at Moorfields, described a pseudo-Argyll Robertson or tonic pupil (Adie's pupil) characterized by a sluggish, prolonged contraction to light; when constricted, the pupil takes an abnormally long time to dilate in darkness or on looking into the distance.

1902   J. O. MCREYNOLDS (1865–1942) of Dallas reported on his pterygium operation to the American Medical Association Section of Ophthalmology. This procedure, which McReynolds popularized, was originated by Desmarres.

1902   BARDIER and CLUZET used a stalagmometer in an attempt to determine the surface tension of aqueous humor.

1902   FÉLIX DE LAPERSONNE in Paris introduced his anterior approach to the levator for the correction of ptosis. This is similar to the current technique.

1902   EMIL C. GRUENING and WILBUR B. MARPLE (b. 1855) of New York City expanded the use of tarsal resection to cases of acquired ptosis.

1903   The distinguished Parisian ophthalmologist LOUIS ÉMILE JAVAL, completely blind from glaucoma since 1900, published *Entre aveugles*, a book of advice to those who are going blind and to their physicians, based on his own experience.

1903   The first volume of the *Encyclopédie française d'ophtalmologie* was published under the editorship of FELIX LAGRANGE of Bordeaux and E. VALUDE of Paris. The ninth and final volume was published in 1910, and the entire work totaled about 8000 pages.

1903   The Western Ophthalmological and Otolaryngological Association was renamed the American Academy of Ophthalmology and Otolaryngology.

1903   LEOPOLD MÜLLER of Vienna suggested a scleral resection operation to reduce the size of the globe in cases of retinal detachment. Müller theorized that stretching of the choroid was the cause of retinal detachment and scleral resection reduced tension on the choroid.

1903   SIR JOHN HERBERT PARSONS of Moorfields published *The ocular circulation* containing the results of his research on that topic.

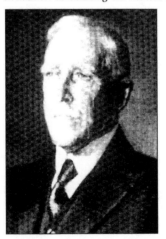

Sir John Herbert Parsons
(1868–1957)

1903	E. KROMPECKER, in *Der Basalzellenkrebs*, contributed the first complete description of a basal cell epithelioma and recognized this tumor to be a carcinoma of basal cells of the epidermis.
1903	CLAUD ALLEY WORTH (1869–1936) of London issued his classic monograph *Squint, its causes and treatment* based on his study of 2337 cases of ocular motility defects. Worth established an orthoptic clinic at Moorfields and introduced a treatment system for children with strabismus.
1903	The first issue of *Transactions of the American Academy of Ophthalmology and Otolaryngology* was distributed to each member of the Academy, containing meeting papers and various proceedings.
1903	WILLIAM L. BALLENGER (1861–1915), an otolaryngologist from Chicago, was elected president of the American Academy of Ophthalmology and Otolaryngology and, together with the ophthalmologists CHRISTIAN R. HOLMES (1857–1920) and DERRICK VAIL (1864–1930), provided the organization with the critical leadership required to assure its success.
1904	ROBERT MARCUS GUNN (1850–1909) of Moorfields discovered the 'Marcus-Gunn' pupil. In this abnormality, when the pupillary activity of one eye is diminished or abolished, the consensual darkness reflex derived from the other eye may dominate the pupillary reactions.

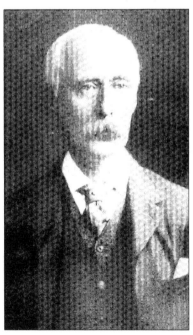

Robert Marcus Gunn
(1850–1909)

1904   H. VON HOFFMANN of Baden Baden gave the first report of conjunctivodacryocystorhinostomy at the Tenth International Congress of Ophthalmology in Lucern. He attached the lacrimal and conjunctival sacs using a buccal mucosa tube.

1904   JULIUS BOLDT, a regimental surgeon in the Prussian army, published *Das Trachoma*. The book gives one of the finest accounts available of the history of trachoma, as well as insights into the challenges ophthalmologists faced before the etiology and effective treatment were discovered.

1904   The Zeiss Optical Company constructed a complicated and elaborate fundus camera for FRIEDRICH DIMMER, then at Graz. The camera was the size of a modern automobile.

1904   ADDEO TOTI (b. 1861) of Florence provided the first modern description of dacryocystorhinostomy by an external approach. Toti exposed the lacrimal sac, resected its inner wall, punched out a corresponding piece of the turbinate bone, resected the corresponding nasal mucous membrane, and sewed up the external wound.

1904   ERNEST MOTAIS was appointed the first ophthalmology professor at the Medical Institute in Angers, France. Motais was an authority on the motor apparatus of the eye and a pioneer in ptosis surgery.

1904   H. V. WÜRDEMANN (1865–1938) of Seattle established the journal *Ophthalmology*. Würdemann also edited the *Annals of Ophthalmology*.

1904   KATE WYLIE BALDWIN, a Philadelphia otolaryngologist, was accepted as the first female member of the American Academy of Ophthalmology and Otolaryngology.

1904   JULES GONIN (1870–1935) of Lausanne, Switzerland published his first report regarding retinal detachment, in which he described three eyes with rhegmatogenous retinal detachment. His study of these specimens and of patients with retinal detachment in his clinic convinced him that a relationship existed between vitreous traction, retinal tears, and retinal detachment.

1904   The American Association of Opticians adopted 'optometrist' and 'optometry' to denote its profession, defining optometry as 'The science which treats of the philosophy of light and sight, and the art of determining the visual status of the human eye and the neutralization of abnormal conditions by lenses.'

1904   JOHN HERBERT PARSONS of London published the first volume of *The pathology of the eye*. The fourth and final volume appeared in 1908.

1904   ARTHUR VON HIPPEL at Königsberg described a disease characterized by capillary angiomas of the retina. The central nervous system component was described by Lindau in 1926.

1905   ISADOR SCHNABEL (1842–1908), a professor in Vienna, proposed a theory on the pathogenesis of glaucoma based on the formation of cavities in front of and behind the lamina cribrosa in eyes with glaucoma (Schnabel's cavernous optic atrophy). He suggested that the glaucomatous cup resulted from the posterior displacement of the lamina into the retrolaminar cavities.

1905   ARMAND TROUSSEAU (1856–1910) of Paris was selected as the director of the Foundation Ophtalmologique Adolphe de Rothschild. Trousseau was noted as a cataract surgeon, and he also studied congenital diseases, iris prolapse, and lacrimal disease. His major work published about this (undated) was *Ophtalmologie: hygiène de l'oeil*.

1905   GEORGE THOMAS STEVENS of New York published *A treatise on the motor apparatus of the eyes*. This book helped to standardize the nomenclature used in strabismus surgery.

1905   HJALMAR AUGUST SCHIÖTZ (1850–1927) of Oslo presented his indentation tonometer for measuring intraocular pressure to the Norwegian Medical Society. This replaced the original mechanical tonometer and remained popular for 50 years.

1905   FRIEDRICH BEST of Dresden published *Über eine hereditäre maculaaffektion*, in which he established that a hereditary feature exists for vitelliform macular dystrophy.

1905   Examination for trachoma was made mandatory for all immigrants arriving in the United States. Those who were found to have the disease were refused entry and sent back to their country of origin.

1905   ERNST FUCHS of Vienna published his landmark article on his pathologic studies of sympathetic ophthalmia. Based on studies of 35 cases, Fuchs described Dalén–Fuchs nodules.

1905   EDWARD JACKSON of Philadelphia and Denver founded *The Ophthalmic Year Book* and was its editor for 24 years.

1905   WILHELM CZERMAK (1856–1906) of Prague modified Krönlein's lateral orbitotomy to obtain wider access to the orbit and leave a more cosmetically satisfactory scar.

1905   The American Academy of Ophthalmology and Otolaryngology recognized itself as an association of two distinct specialties and segregated the presentations at its annual meeting into an otologic section and an ophthalmology section that ran concurrently.

1905   CAVAZZANI initiated his studies to determine the viscosity of aqueous humor. He completed his work in 1909.

1906   SANTIAGO RAMÓN Y CAJAL, neurohistologist of Madrid, who contributed the classic account of the vertebrate retina, was awarded the Nobel Prize.

1906   SIR CHARLES SCOTT SHERRINGTON, physiologist at Liverpool and Oxford, published: 'On the proprio-ceptive system, especially in its reflex action' in *Brain* and *The integrative action of the nervous system*. Sherrington's experimental studies on reflex action had a profound influence on modern ophthalmic physiology.

1906   The AMA and the American Academy of Ophthalmology and Otolaryngology proposed legislation to control ophthalmia neonatorum through the education of practitioners and midwives, the registration of midwives, and compulsory reporting of all cases.

1906   JULES GONIN of Lausanne attributed retinal tears to vitreoretinal adhesions in a chapter on diseases of the retina written with his professor, MARC DUFOUR. This appeared in the *Encyclopédie française d'ophtalmologie*.

1906   EDUARD KONRAD ZIRM (1887–1944) of Olomouc, Czechoslovakia performed the first successful penetrating keratoplasty using fresh human tissue. Despite the success, lamellar grafts maintained their popularity for the next 20 years.

1906   CHARLES CONRAD MILLER (1881–1950) of Chicago published the first article devoted solely to cosmetic aspects of 'bag-like folds of eye skin.' He proposed an operation using cocaine infiltration for anesthesia to remove crescents of wrinkled skin.

1906   ALLVAR GULLSTRAND, professor of ophthalmology in Uppsala, stated that the yellow color of the macula lutea is a cadaveric phenomenon.

1906   LUCIEN HOWE of Buffalo wrote his authoritative two-volume work *Muscles of the eye*, in which he elucidates the problems of ocular motility.

1907   EDWARD JACKSON of Denver published an article proposing the use of crossed cylinders to measure the astigmatic axes and the ocular cylindrical error.

1907   THEODOR AXENFELD, professor of ophthalmology at Freiburg, published *Die Bakteriologie in der Augenheilkunde*. This book followed the format of VICTOR MORAX'S earlier chapter on conjuctival infection in the *Encyclopédie française d'ophtalmologie*.

1907   WILHELM CZERMAK of Prague published the authoritative *Augenärztlichen operationen*.

1907	ERNEST EDMUND MADDOX of Edinburgh invented the 'Maddox prism verger' for ocular motility testing.
1907	LUCIEN HOWE of Buffalo published *Muscles of the eye*, a landmark contribution to the topic of ocular motility.
1907	FRIEDRICH DIMMER from the University of Vienna demonstrated his improved method of photographing the ocular fundus in *Die Photographie des Augenhitergrundes*, a synopsis of his work on fundus photography.
1907	CHARLES CONRAD MILLER of Chicago published *Cosmetic surgery: the correction of featural imperfections*. This was the first book devoted entirely to cosmetic surgery.
1907	Piper invented the electromyograph, which facilitated the study of the rapidity and intensity of contraction and relaxation of ocular muscles.
1907	The American Academy of Ophthalmology and Otolaryngology with 434 members had grown into the largest specialty medical society in the United States.
1907	LUDWIG HALBERSTAEDTER (b. 1876) and STANISLAUS VON PROWAZEK (1875–1915) found infectious inclusion bodies in pus cells from eyes with trachoma.
1908	EDWARD NETTLESHIP identified the autosomal recessive inheritance pattern in his study of nearly 1000 families with retinal degenerations.
1908	COLONEL HENRY SMITH of the Punjab demonstrated his 'Smith-Indian' cataract technique in the United States and England. His method was difficult to perform and had a high rate of vitreous loss.
1908	The US Public Health Service discovered trachoma among inhabitants of the Appalachian Mountains in eastern Kentucky. Prior to that time trachoma was not considered an American problem.
1908	A bill was passed in New York state regulating optometry and establishing its professionalization. This followed twelve years of lobbying by optometrists and led to the creation of the Optical Society of the State of New York.
1908	*The eye and the nervous system*, edited by WILLIAM CAMPBELL POSEY (1866–1934), a Philadelphia ophthalmologist, and WILLIAM GIBSON SPILLER (1863–1940), a Philadelphia neurologist, was published. This was the first American book to focus solely on neuro-ophthalmology.
1908	GEORGE COATS (1876–1915), curator of pathology at Moorfields, reported on 'Forms of retinal disease with massic exudation,'

including 23 photographic plates. That disorder, originally called retinitis circinata, is now known as Coats' disease.

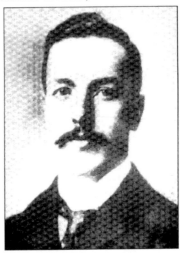

George Coats
(1876–1915)

1908   THEODOR LEBER in Heidelberg, after extensive experience examining retinal detachments under the microscope, concluded that retinal tears were a secondary event caused by extensive preretinal organization.

1908   JOSEF MELLER (b. 1874) wrote *Ophthalmic surgery* as a companion to Ernst Fuchs's lectures at the Second Eye Clinic in Vienna. This book was particularly popular with Americans, and updated editions continued to appear until 1953.

1908   VLADIMIR PETROVICH FILATOV (1875–1956) of Odessa completed his 400-page dissertation on the 'Study of the toxic action of cells in ophthalmology.'

1909   ROBERT HENRY ELLIOT (1866–1936), of the British Indian Medical Service, described his corneoscleral trephining procedure for open-angle glaucoma. Elliot split the cornea to avoid the ciliary body. It resulted in a large success rate, but a serious complication was hypotony.

1909   E. PAYR (1882–1967) in Germany significantly improved the ptosis correction technique of frontalis suspension by introducing the use of a single central sling of fascia lata.

1909   KARL STARGARDT (1875–1927) of Marburg gave the first report of a recessively inherited macular dystrophy, commonly referred to as Stargardt disease.

1909   *The Journal of the National Medical Association* was established, and

CHARLES VICTOR ROMAN served as the first editor.

1909   TATSUJI INOUYE (1880–1976) of Tokyo published *Die Sehstörungen bein Schussverletzungen der kortikalen Sehsphäre, nach Beobachtungen an Verwundenten der letzten japanischen Kriege*. This outlined Inouye's study of soldiers with visual field loss caused by cerebral lesions.

1909   S. LEWIS ZIEGLER (1861–1926) of Philadelphia repopularized cautery for the treatment of ectropion and entropion.

1909   PAUL EHRLICH (1858–1915) of Berlin introduced the use of salvarsan (arsenobenzol) in preventing and treating syphilitic disease in the eye and elsewhere. Salvarsan was noted to cause severe collateral effects on the eye and nervous system.

1909   CASEY ALBERT WOOD at Northwestern University reported a surgical technique for excising the thickened membrane from the bottom of the nasolacrimal duct in congenital nasolacrimal duct obstruction using a small trochar canula and obturator. In the same year Wood published his *System of ophthalmic therapeutics*. He includes a short chapter on venesection.

1909   J. C. BERRY independently reported a technique for the treatment of congenital nasolacrimal duct obstruction in the *Boston Medical and Surgical Journal* that involved the use of a cutting-edge forceps to remove the membrane from the nasolacrimal duct.

1909   The American Association of Opticians created the National Board of State Examiners in Optometry. The following year the Association changed its name to the American Optical Association.

1909   EDWARD NETTLESHIP reported on his important investigations into the role of heredity in night blindness, retinitis pigmentosa, albinis, and other eye diseases. Nettleship and C. H. Usher are considered the founders of ophthalmic genetics in England.

1910   HENRY MEIGE, a French neurologist, gave the first description of blepharospasm, which he termed 'spasm facial median.' Meige had a strong interest in tics, gesticulations, and related movement disorders.

1910   COLONEL HENRY SMITH of the British Indian Medical Service published *The treatment of cataract*. This presented the 'Smith-Indian' method of intracapsular cataract extraction, which he had employed in over 24,000 extractions.

1910   J. M. WEST, an otolaryngologist at Johns Hopkins Medical School, was the first to devise an endonasal or internal approach to dacryocystorhinostomy. West removed the mucosa over the lacrimal protuberances as well as a portion of the ascending ramus of the maxilla and lacrimal bone. After exposing the lacrimal sac, the nasal wall of the sac was excised.

1910 The *Practical Optician*, a journal for optometrists, was founded. It has undergone several name changes and is published today under the title *The Optometric Weekly*.

1910 CHARLES HEADY BEARD (1855–1916) of Chicago published his *Ophthalmic surgery*, the most comprehensive English-language ophthalmic surgery text of its time.

1910 Oxford University instituted a diploma for the ophthalmology specialty at the urgings of ROBERT WALTER DOYNE, senior surgeon at Oxford Eye Hospital.

1910 DERRICK T. VAIL, professor of ophthalmology in Cincinatti, at the Academy meeting presented a paper and gave a detailed lantern slide demonstration of the Smith-Indian technique of cataract surgery.

1910 ABRAHAM FLEXNER (1866–1959) published the 'Flexner Report' on medical education in the USA and Canada. The report led to widespread reform in US and Canadian medical education and the closure of over 50% of white medical schools and over 75% of black medical schools.

1910 SAMUEL ERNEST WHITNALL (1876–1950), a prosector at Oxford, published his description of the 'superior transverse ligament.'

1911 ANDRÉ MAGITOT of Paris published a report of a corneal lamellar homograft that remained clear for a year after surgery. In the same year he made the observation that corneal tissue could be preserved for at least several days prior to use.

1911 ALLVAR GULLSTRAND, professor of physiologic optics at the University of Uppsala, received the Nobel Prize for his simplified mathematical model of the optics of the human eye. In the same year, he developed an optic imagery system based on his model that allowed the development of both an ophthalmoscope fundus camera and slit-lamp biomicroscope that was free of reflections from the patient's cornea and lens.

1911 FREDERICK STRANGE COLLE (1871–1929), a New York plastic surgeon, described and illustrated a surgical method for excising wrinkled skin from the eyelids in his *Plastic and cosmetic surgery*. He was the first to describe the importance of marking the skin preoperatively to determine the amount of skin to be removed.

1911 J. DOLLINGER in Germany gave the initial report of orbital decompression for endocrine exophthalmos using Krönlein's lateral orbitotomy approach.

1911   ADDEO TOTI of Florence realized that when a dacryocystorhinostomy was unsuccessful, it was usually the result of too small a bony window; he recommended that the size of the opening be increased.

1911   JOHANNES OHM (b. 1880) in Germany introduced the injection of air into the vitreous cavity as a method for retinal reattachment treatment.

1911   G. F. KEIPER addressed the subject of cataract surgeries in elderly patients at the American Academy of Ophthalmology and Otolaryngology meeting. Surgery was considered dangerous for aged patients because of the risk of delirium, prostatic obstruction, and pulmonary problems caused by the prolonged forced bed rest with both eyes bandaged. Keiper noted that a survey of 300 ophthalmologists revealed that seven patients over the age of 100, all women, had undergone cataract surgery.

1911   SAMUEL ERNEST WHITNALL at Oxford described the insertion of the lateral canthal tendon into the lateral orbital tubercle and the relationship between the lacrimal fossa and the ethmoidal air cells.

1912   ROBERT HENRY ELLIOT of Madras published his paper 'Sclerocorneal trephining in the operative treatment of glaucoma.'

1912   The American Medical Association revised its initial code of ethics into the Principles of Medical Ethics. The foundation of the code rested on the Hippocratic Corpus and Thomas Percival's *Medical Ethics*.

1912   LASZLO DE BLASKOVICS (1869–1938) of Budapest introduced lamellar scleral resection in the treatment of retinal detachment.

1912   ANTON ELSCHNIG (1863–1939) of Prague reported an effective treatment for involutional ectropion using an eyelid skin flap. This was accomplished by means of a medial-plasty incision with the upper and lower arms of the Z following the natural lid contour.

1912   MAXIMILIAN SALZMANN (1862–1954), professor of ophthalmology at

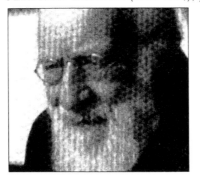

Maximilian Salzmann
(1862–1954)

the University of Graz, published *Anatomy and histology of the human eyeball in its normal state: Its development and senescence*. This was one of the final textbooks in histology to use drawings rather than photographs. Salzmann's description of the anterior chamber angle was among the earliest to be accurate.

1912   STEPHEN L. POLYAK (1889–1955) of Chicago advocated an endonasal approach for dacryocystorhinostomy.

1912   The intracapsular cataract extraction technique of GEORGHE STANCULEANU (1874–1918) of Bucharest was presented to the American Academy of Ophthalmology and Otolaryngology. The operation consisted of detaching the zonalar fibers of the anterior capsule using forceps and extracting the lens with pressure applied by a spoon.

1912   ERNEST EDMUND MADDOX of Edinburgh designed the 'Maddox wing test' for ocular motility testing.

1912   VLADIMIR PETROVICH FILATOV of Odessa began his work on corneal transplantation. He initially used a donor cornea with a narrow rim of sclera. The undermined conjuctiva was sewn in a pursestring over the donor's periphery. This was tried in two cases, both of which failed.

1913   SIR CHARLES SCOTT SHERRINGTON was appointed professor of physiology at Oxford. Over the next 23 years, he created what was to be considered the best school of physiology in the world. Many of the researches carried out were relevant to ophthalmology.

1913   E. HERTEL of Leipzig gave the first report of hyperosmotic agent treatment that resulted in a short-term decrease of IOP.

1913   The U.S. Public Health Service began a campaign to eradicate trachoma—despite not knowing the causative microbial agent—among Appalachian Mountain residents in eastern Kentucky. Treatment consisted of sanitation, hygiene, and nutrition.

1913   DAVID HARROWER of Worcester, Massachusetts exhibited before the American Ophthalmological Society an electric Morton-Marple ophthalmoscope powered by a two-cell battery that was screwed into the instrument. Harrower called the illumination mechanism simple, cheap, and effective.

1913   Novocaine was first used by BALFOUR for nerve-block anesthesia.

1913   The first volume of *The American encyclopedia of ophthalmology* was published under the editorial supervision of CASEY ALBERT WOOD, professor of ophthalmology at Northwestern University. More than 100 ophthalmologists contributed, and publication of the subsequent 17 volumes continued until 1921.

1913   Fredrich H. Verhoeff of Boston reintroduced C. R. Agnew's conjunctival incision for drainage of the lacrimal sac made through the conjuctiva between the caruncle and inner commissure of the eyelids, and Verhoeff then dilated the nasolacrimal duct with lacrimal probes. Verhoeff, in the same year, proposed an eyelid skin flap procedure to correct involutional ectroption. He advocated the use of a suture along with two shirt buttons to support the lower lid. His operation allowed for the lid tension to be adjusted during the first two weeks until permanent fibrosis fixed the lid in the desired position.

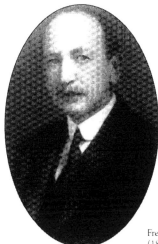

Frederick Hermann Verhoeff
(1874–1968)

1913   Pennsylvania optometrists sued to prevent the inclusion of ocular refraction study under an umbrella regulation of the practice of medicine. The judge's decision in favor of the optometrists, ruled that optometry was 'separate and distinct' from medicine.

1913   The American Board for Ophthalmic Examinations was founded through the joint actions of the American Academy of Ophthalmology and Otolaryngology, the AMA's Section on Ophthalmology, and the American Ophthalmological Society.

1914   Clt. Usher in England found autosomal recessive disease to be the most common inheritance pattern in his study of 41 families with retinal degeneration.

1914   Maximilian Salzmann of Vienna, generally considered the founder of gonioscopy, published two fundamental works on the angle of the anterior chamber that provided the basis for gonioscopy. In order to get a clearer picture of the angle, he made use of a contact lens invented by Adolf Fick. Included in his work were drawings of the angle and its abnormalities, including blood filling the canal of Schlemm.

1914   AUGUST VAN LINT (1877–1959) of Brussels introduced orbicularis muscle akinesia for cataract extraction.

1914   DeZENG of Camden, New Jersey began manufacturing an ophthalmoscope with two batteries in the handle and a round-glass perforated mirror. This instrument remained popular for the succeeding two decades.

1914   CHARLES HENRY MAY introduced an electric ophthalmoscope that had separate discs containing concave and convex lenses and substituted a solid glass prism for the mirror. Its handle enclosed a small electric bulb and battery. Bausch & Lomb manufactured this ophthalmoscope, and it enjoyed wide popularity for more than 50 years.

1914   The American Optical Association recommended that operators of motor vehicles, still relatively rare, be required to pass visual examinations.

1914   CHARLES HEADY BEARD of Chicago authored a chapter entitled 'Semeiology and diagnosis,' for *International system of ophthalmic practice*. His beautiful drawings of the fundus were admired and awarded a diploma from the American Medical Association.

1914   HERMANN KUHNT of Bonn improved Addeo Toti's dacryocystorhinostomy operation by suturing flaps of the nasal mucosa to the periosteum to limit the formation of granulation tissue.

1914   ANTON ELSCHNIG of Prague reported his first successful result in penetrating keratoplasty in a patient with interstitial keratitis. The graft was 4 mm in diameter and had been excised with a von Hippel trephine. It was held in place by the pressure of the lids and five years postoperatively was in part transparent. The patient's vision was reported at 0.6 to 0.7.

1915   The original WELCH-ALLYN ophthalmoscope was patented by MR. WILLIAM N. ALLYN of Skaneateles, New York. The lightbulb was attached to the face of the instrument, eliminating the need for a reflecting system.

1915   To improve educational standards for optometrists, the American Optical Association officially recommended minimum requirements of two 26-week terms of study.

1915   The American Academy of Ophthalmology and Otolaryngology established a Commission on the Etiology of Iritis, which surveyed case histories of iritis to determine the causes of the disorder. The

Academy also funded research at the New York Eye and Ear Infirmary for this purpose.

1915 The National Committee for the Prevention of Blindness with offices in New York was formed by a merger of the American Association for the Conservation of Vision (1910) and the New York State Committee for the Prevention of Blindness (1913). All of these organizations were involved in investigating the question of blindness from ophthalmia neonatorum.

1916 THEODOR LEBER in Heidelberg theorized that retinal and pigment epithelial degeneration was the cause of retinitis pigmentosa.

1916 O. HENKER combined the Czapski corneal microscope with the GULLSTRAND illuminating unit. ALFRED VOGT subsequently added an adjustable slit to the lamp, allowing for variable methods of illumination. By combining a microscope with slit-lamp illumination, it became possible to study the histology of the living eye with a diagnostic tool second in importance only to the ophthalmoscope.

1916 BIRCH-HIRSCHFELD in Königsberg introduced the transposition of the orbicularis muscle to correct involutional ectropion.

1916 FREDRICK H. VERHOEFF of Boston introduced the use of conjunctivoscleral sutures to close the cataract wound.

1916 The first certification examination in an American medical specialty was administered by the American Board of Ophthalmic Examination on December 13 and 14 at the University of Tennessee College of Medicine in Memphis. Ophthalmology was thus the first medical specialty to establish standardized testing for competence.

1916 J. W. MILLETTE recommended at the American Academy of Ophthalmology and Otolaryngology meeting that binocular surgical bandages not be used after cataract surgery. This was a change from past recommendations of leaving the dressings on for at least several days following the procedure. Millette also advocated quicker ambulation.

1916 SHINOBU ISHIHARA (1879–1963) of Japan published *Test for Colour-Blindness* a set of colored plates that Ishihara developed to test the color vision of military recruits when the Stilling color vision charts proved inadequate.

1916 HENRICUS JACOBUS MARIA WEBE (1888–1961) was appointed chief ophthalmologist in Rotterdam and wrote 'Keratitus urica,' which dealt with various forms of gouty eye disease.

1917 WILLIAM LEMUEL BENEDICT (1885–1969) was appointed head of the Section of Ophthalmology at the Mayo Clinic. He had an illustrious

185

career and made important contributions to the literature on tumors of the orbit, among other topics.

1917   CASEY ALBERT WOOD of Chicago, ophthalmologist and ornithologist, published his classic *Fundus oculi of birds*.

1917   ANDRÉ MAGITOT of Paris challenged Leber's conclusion that the aqueous humor is produced by transudation from the ciliary body and has a primary circulation. Magitot maintains there is little or no flow of fluid but rather a general interchange through the tissues of the eye.

1917   PAUL BAILLART (1877–1969) of Paris introduced the first ophthalmodynamometer of acceptable sensitivity to measure the relationships between the intraocular pressure and the systolic pressure in the central retinal artery.

1917   FÉLIX LAGRANGE, professor of ophthalmology at the University of Bordeaux, issued his monograph on orbital fractures. This work included a detailed historical summary of the diagnosis and treatment of orbital fractures.

1917   The US Surgeon General's Office established a military eye, ear, nose, and throat hospital in France staffed by American ophthalmologists and otolaryngologists.

1917   *The British Journal of Ophthalmology* began publication. This was an amalgamation of several journals, including *Ophthalmic Review*, *Reports of the Ophthalmic Hospital*, and *Ophthalmoscope*.

1917   The American Board of Ophthalmic Examinations established standardized examinations, which were held in New York City and Pittsburgh, following the trial run in Memphis in 1916. Candidates could, however, bypass the examination based on their previous experience in ophthalmology, and only one-third of the initial 120 recipients of the certificate actually passed the exam.

1917   IGNACIO BARRAQUER (1884–1965) demonstrated his erisiphake for cataract extraction.

1918   HEINRICH LEOPOLD SCHOELER (1844–1918), professor of ophthalmology in Berlin, introduced the use of a freezing technique to produce a chorioretinal scar in cases of retinal detachment. He did this by the application of carbonic snow to the sclera.

1918   THOMAS HALL SHASTID (1866–1947) of St. Louis provided the first English translation of Helmholtz's *Beischriebung eines Augen—Spiegels* (*Description of an eye-speculum for the examination of the retina of the living eye*).

1918   The *American Journal of Ophthalmology* began publication of its 'third series,' absorbing the *Ophthalmic Record, Annals of Ophthalmology,* and *Ophthalmic Year Book.*

1918   JOHANNES F. S. ESSER (1877–1946) of Holland described a full-thickness skin graft technique utilizing an arterialized pedicicle flap to reconstruct the lower lid, which he termed a 'biological flap.'

1918   JULES GONIN of Lausanne presented a paper to the Swiss Ophthalmological Society in which he supported his thesis that ideopathic retinal tears were caused by vitreous traction and were the source of retinal detachments. He cited the previously published theories of Leber and Nordenson and hypothesized that vitreo-retinal adhesions were the result of equatorial and preequatorial foci of chorioretinitis.

1918   EDWARD TREACHER COLLINS of Moorfields and M. STEPHEN MAYOU (b. 1876) collaborated to produce an important pathology and microbiology text, *Pathology and bacteriology of the eye.*

1918   ARNOLD KNAPP (1869–1956), director of the Herman Knapp Memorial Eye Hospital in New York City, published his influential *Medical ophthalmology.*

1919   JULES GONIN of Lausanne presented to the Swiss Ophthalmological Society his initial surgical successes repairing retinal tears involving combined drainage of subretinal fluid with direct treatment of the break by transscleral cautery.

1919   The American Optical Association was renamed the American Optometric Association.

1919   LEONARD KOEPPE (1884–1969) of the University of Berlin contributed to the development of gonioscopy as a clinical method of examination by offering an alternative to the Czapski binocular microscope.

1920   Trachoma was recognized as a significant problem in the Middle East, affecting an estimated 60% of Arab school children in Syria, Lebanon, and Palestine and 90% of the population in Egypt.

1920   E. J. CURRAN of Kansas City theorized that angle closure was caused by aqueous humor trapped in the posterior chamber and that a shallow anterior chamber was due to the iris protruding frontward. Curan attributed the curative effect of Graefe's iridectomy in acute glaucoma to reestablishing the free passage of aqueous from the posterior to the anterior chamber.

1920   JOHANNES OHM improved ADDEO TOTI'S operation for dacryocystorhinostomy by suturing the margins of the nasal mucosa to the lacrimal sac.

1920   O. BAUM, a Prague physician, reported that he had produced herpetic keratitis in rabbit corneas by injecting vesicular fluid from cases of herpes labialis and herpes genitalis.

1920   Archaeologists discovered a statue depicting an oculist in the pyramid of Giza.

1920   JULES GONIN of Lausanne reported to the French Ophthalmology Society his success in curing several cases of retinal detachment. His operation consisted of localization of the retinal break followed by closure of the break by transscleral thermocauterization, deliberately perforating the sclera and allowing the subretinal fluid to escape.

1920   MÜLLER proposed the 'halving' technique (a carpentry principle which he applied to correct eyelid notching) to correct involutional ectropion.

1921   ANDRÉ MAGITOT and PAUL BAILLART of Paris reported their findings on the relative roles of the retinal and uveal vessels in the nutrition of the retina. In the same year Magitot and MESTREZAT published their findings on the chemical profile of the aqueous humor.

1921   OTTO BARKAN (1887–1958), trained in ophthalmology in Vienna and Munich, returned to his birthplace of San Francisco, where he focused on understanding the causative mechanism and treatment of glaucoma.

1921   J. W. TUDOR THOMAS (1893–1976) from Cardiff, Wales successfully transplanted 50 corneas among animals of the same species. Thomas concluded that successful grafts could only be achieved using tissue from the same species.

1921   The Registry of Ophthalmic Pathology, begun largely through the efforts of HARRY SEARLS GRADLE (1883–1950), allowed the Academy members to provide pathological materials while the Army Medical Museum provided the technical staff for the preparation of specimens and a facility to house the Academy's collection.

1920   FREDERICK WILLIAM EDRIDGE-GREEN of London published *Physiology of vision*, which described his studies of how many colors people typically see (he claimed six or seven) and his elaborate theory of color vision. He developed a pocket wool-test and lantern test for color blindness.

1921   ERNEST EDMUND MADDOX delivered his classic Doyne lecture on the 'heterophorias.'

1921   *The anatomy of the human orbit and accessory organs of vision* was published by SAMUEL ERNEST WHITNALL, the chair of anatomy at Bristol. This presented the anatomical information needed to perform competent ophthalmic surgery. Whitnall also published numerous articles describing orbital topographic anatomy.

1921   JOHN MARTIN WHEELER (1879–1938) of New York City, a founder of ophthalmic plastic surgery, proposed a flap graft of skin from the upper eyelid inferiorly to support the lower lid in a superior-posterior direction to correct involutional ectropion.

1921   LOUIS DUPUY-DUTEMPS (1871–1946) with JULIEN BOURGUET (1876–1952) of Paris described a technique of external dacryocystorhinostomy, which involved incising the posterior wall of the lacrimal sac without removal of tissue, and subsequent anastomosis of the lacrimal and nasal mucosa so that no wound edges would remain to scar. They reported a cure rate of 95% in 1000 cases using this method. This firmly established external dacryocystorhinostomy as an accepted method.

1921   HARRY SEARLS GRADLE was appointed to the faculty at the University of Illinois College of Medicine, where he became an expert in glaucoma and was a leader in developing instruction courses and home study courses for the American Academy of Ophthalmology and Otolaryngology.

1921   ALFRED VOGT (1879–1943) of Zurich published *Lehrbuch und Atlas der Spaltlampen-mikroskopie des lebenden Auges*. This single-volume atlas contains many of the observations he made while using the slit-lamp biomicroscope to study a vast spectrum of eye conditions of the anterior segment.

1921   The American Optical Company patented an instrument called the Lensometer designed to accurately measure lens power with light.

1921   S. LEWIS ZEIGLER (1861–1926) of Philadelphia advocated total discission for the removal of congenital cataract in those under the age of ten. Linear extraction was recommended for older children.

1922   ROBERT HENRY ELLIOT of Madras published *Treatise on glaucoma* that further popularized his trephining procedure for glaucoma.

1922   FREDERICK VERHOEFF was appointed the principal consultant in ophthalmology pathology for the Registry of Ophthalmic Pathology. Major George Russell Callender was the in-house pathologist, and other consulting ophthalmic pathologists included Harry Searls Gradle of Chicago, Jonas Friedenwald of Baltimore, and Georgiana Dvorak Theobald of Chicago.

1922   SCHOTT put two electrodes of a string galvanometer on either side of the eye to study the electrophysiology of contraction and the relaxation of ocular muscles.

1922   LASZLO DE BLASKOVICS, professor of ophthalmology in Budapest, proposed a levator resection method for the treatment of ptosis using a refined conjunctival approach. This method is still in use today.

1923   FRITZ PREGL, an Austrian ophthalmologist, was awarded the Nobel Prize for chemistry for his methodology for microanalysis of organic substances.

1923   CLAUDE MONET, the impressionist painter, underwent cataract surgery after he was forced to stop painting by his loss of vision. Three years after his first surgery, Monet resumed painting.

1923   ADALBERT FUCHS (1887–1973) of Vienna, son of Ernst Fuchs, published *Atlas der Histopathologie des Auges*, an important text on ophthalmic pathology.

1923   P. LAMOINE and G. VOLOIS viewed the 'posterior segment' of the eye by using a binocular corneal microscope in combination with a concave lens and diffuse illumination.

1923   The Ophthalmological Society of the United Kingdom recognized the Philadelphia ophthalmologist GEORGE EDMUND DE SCHWEINITZ's many accomplishments by selecting him as the first American to give the Bowman lecture, 'Certain ocular aspects of pituitary body disorders.'

1924   HENRY P. WAGENER (1890–1961) published his initial observations on hypertensive retinopathy, which ultimately became known as the Keith-Wagener-Barker classification (*Archives of Internal Medicine*).

1924   RUDOLPH THIEL (1894–1967) of Frankfurt am Main proposed the use of sympatholytic drugs for the treatment of glaucoma.

1924   VAN CREVELD used a torsion balance to estimate the surface tension of aqueous humor.

1924   CARL HENRY ZEISS (1877–1961) produced the first slit lamp based on Alvar Gullstrand's ophthalmoscope and designed by Nordenson that was relatively compact, eliminated most light reflexes, and used carbon arc illumination.

1924   JULIEN BOURGUET of Paris described a surgical approach for the removal of herniated intraorbital fat through the mucosa of the conjunctival cul-de-sac of the lower eyelid. In the same year, he published the first cosmetic blepharoplasty article to include pictures of patients taken before and after surgery.

1925   EDMUND BENJAMIN SPAETH (1890–1976) of Philadelphia published one of the first English language oculoplastics books, *Newer methods of ophthalmic plastic surgery*.

1925   H. L. AMOS and coworkers demonstrated that herpetic disease was caused by a virus.

1925   DIETER used a capillary viscometer to more accurately determine the viscosity of the aqueous humor.

1925   GEORGIANA DVORAK-THEOBALD was appointed chief pathologist at Cook County Hospital. She was noted most for her work on the lens capsule and the anatomy of the canal of Schlemm.

1925   HARRY SEARLS GRADLE of Chicago introduced the use of epinephrine as treatment for glaucoma. Epinephrine was enthusiastically used until the adverse side effect of acute glaucoma was reported. Subsequently, it was not considered a safe drug for the treatment of glaucoma until the 1940s, when gonioscopy permitted ophthalmologists to distinguish narrow-angle eyes that would be adversely affected by epinephrine therapy.

1925   The American Optometric Association newsletter *AOA Messenger* was first published.

1926   EDMUND BENJAMIN SPAETH proposed his 'rotated island graft operation' for pterygium.

1926   The American Ophthalmologic Society adapted the term 'retinoblastoma' as suggested by Verhoeff to be used instead of 'glioma of the retina' to designate the retinal tumor of infants and children.

1926   ARVID LINDAU, a Swedish pathologist, described angiomatosis of the central nervous system and recognized its association with the angiomas of the retina von Hippel described in 1904.

1926   A. SUZANNE NOËL of Paris published *La chirurgie esthétique: son rôle social*. She was a pioneer in producing photographic documentation as an integral part of the practice of cosmetic ophthalmic plastic surgery.

1926   HERMENGILDO ARRUGA (1886–1972) of Barcelona contributed his thesis on 'A simplified modification of the dacryocystorhinostomy.'

1927   HARRY MOSS TRAQUAIR (1875–1954) of Edinburgh published *An introduction to clinical perimetry* that focused on tangent screen campimetry. He described a great number of field defects occurring in ocular and neurological diseases, as well as the technique of tangent screen testing.

1927   SIR W. STEWART DUKE-ELDER (1898–1978) published *Recent advances in ophthalmology*, in which he attempted to show the impact of new discoveries in chemistry and physics on ophthalmology.

1927   J. EASTMAN SHEEHAN of New York published *Plastic surgery of the orbit*, one of the earliest textbooks devoted to orbital surgery. Sheehan favored the use of ear cartilage as a tarsal replacement in lid reconstruction.

1927   T. THORBURN of Sweden published his dissertation on peripheral anterior iris synechiae (PAS) in glaucoma based on the examination of 90 eyes. He was the first to photograph the angle and determined that most eyes with primary glaucoma have open angles.

1927   LUTHER C. PETER (1869–1942), professor of ophthalmology at Temple University in Philadelphia, published *The extra-ocular muscles; a clinical study of normal and abnormal ocular motility.*

1927   JONAS S. FRIEDENWALD wrote *The pathology of the eye,* published in 1929. This was based on a series of lectures given to Johns Hopkins medical students and formed 'a bridge' leading from general pathology to ophthalmic pathology.

1927   BOTHMAN and COHEN used injections of adrenalin to constrict the retinal arteries of rabbits.

1927   ARNOLD PILLAT (1891–1975) of Vienna coauthored with FRIEDRICH DIMMER, who died in 1926, an atlas of fundus photographs taken with the fundus camera the Zeiss Optical Company constructed for Dimmer in 1904.

1927   MAUNO VANNAS (1891–1965) in Helsinki wrote 'Clinical studies about the effect of adrenalin in glaucoma.' This preceded by 30 years the widespread use of epinephrine in the treatment of this disease.

1928   The American Medical Association took over publication of the *Archives of Ophthalmology,* continuing ARNOLD KNAPP as editor.

1928   ERNEST EDMUND MADDOX of Edinburgh developed the 'duochrome test' for near vision testing.

1928   GEORGE S. DERBY (1875–1931) of Harvard advanced blepharoptosis surgery by positioning a single sling from the central tarsus to the upper lateral and medial eyebrow border.

1928   DAME IDA CAROLINE MANN published *The development of the human eye* based on the work she carried out with W. ERNEST FRAZER of the University of London. In the same year, Mann was selected the Doyne Memorial Lecturer by the Ophthalmological Society of the United Kingdom.

1928   MARC AMSLER (1891–1968) at Lausanne developed a test chart (Amsler grid) used to detect retinal abnormalities.

1928   JOSEPH IMRE JR. (1884–1945) in Bratislava, Hungary proposed a tongue-shaped flap from the mid-lower eyelid superiorly and medially to correct involutional ectropion.

Dame Ida Caroline Mann
(1893–1983)

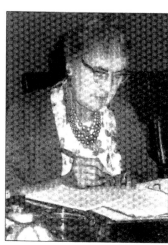

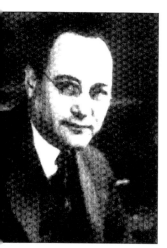

Jonas S. Friedenwald
(1897–1955)

Georgiana Dvorak-Theobold
(1884–1971)

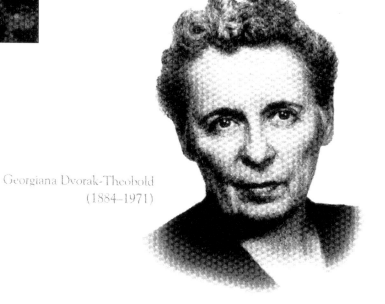

1928   JONAS S. FRIEDENWALD at the Wilmer Institute designed a 'giant' ophthalmoscope to include a wide range or brightness of light intensity, allowing for a more detailed examination of the fundus, particularly through hazy media.

1928   MYER WEINER (1876–1965) of St. Louis proposed an operation for involutional ectropion in which the lower lid was supported with a fascia lata sling anchored at respective canthi.

1928   The National Society for the Prevention of Blindness was formed through the amalgamation of several societies.

1928   ARNOLD KNAPP of New York City addressed the American Academy of Ophthalmology and Otolaryngology on the best method of cataract extraction. He concluded that there was no ideal method and recommended that intracapsular cataract extraction be performed only in selected cases.

1928   KARL WESSELY of Munich began editing the ophthalmic section of 'Henke-Lubarsch,' an important reference work replete with information fundamental to pathology. When completed in 1937, this section (volume 11) totaled 2200 pages, including extensive contributions by Von Hippel, Greef, Elschnig, von Szily, and others.

1928   SIR ALEXANDER FLEMING (1881–1955), a British bacteriologist, discovered penicillin. It was not until the 1950s that this became available to physicians and became the standard treatment for ophthalmia neonatorum, ocular syphilis, and other eye infections.

1929   CECIL S. O'BRIEN (1898–1977) in Iowa City described nerve-block anesthesia of the facial nerve. His technique consisted of injection of anesthetic over the exit of the facial nerve as it crosses the condyloid process in front of the ear.

1929   The American Optometric Association journal *AOA Organizer* was begun. The following year it was renamed the *Journal of the American Optometric Association*.

1929   EDGAR DOUGLAS ADRIAN (1889–1977) at Cambridge and DETLEV WULF BRONK (1897–1975) introduced the use of needle electrodes to measure the intensity and rapidity of ocular muscle contractions.

1929   JONAS S. FRIEDENWALD of Baltimore published his findings regarding methyl alcohol blindness and concluded that ingestion of methyl alcohol led to widespread destruction of the optic nerve.

1929   VICTOR MORAX and PAUL PETIT, both in Paris, coauthored *La trachome*, the culmination of over 30 years of studying trachoma.

1929   EMIL GROSZ (1865–1941) of Budapest was elected chair of the

International League Against Trachoma. This organization stressed the importance of the eradication of trachoma and initiated other organizations and journals devoted to achieving this end.

1929   The importance of JULES GONIN'S work on his ignipuncture surgery was recognized during the International Congress of Ophthalmology in Amsterdam. Following the conference, many ophthalmologists visited Gonin to observe his retinal detachment surgery.

1929   ARTHUR BEDELL (1879–1973) of Albany published his superb atlas of black-and-white fundus photographs.

1930   HENRICUS JACOBUS MARIA WEBE of Utrecht described the use of surface diathermy in retinal detachment surgery. This method allowed for better regulation of intensity and permitted the treatment of an extensive area of the sclera.

1930   The introduction of photographic film in place of glass plates and electronic flash in place of carbon arc illumination add to the versatility of fundus cameras.

1930   ALFRED VOGT of Zurich published the first volume of his three-volume *Atlas der Spaltlampenmikroskopie des Leibenden Auges*, laying the foundation for a new branch of ophthalmology, slit-lamp biomicroscopy. The final volume appeared in 1932.

1930   The National Institute of Health in Bethesda, Maryland, was established by the United States Congress to administer medical research programs conducted by the Public Health Service.

1930   ADOLPH FRANCESCHETTI (1896–1966), while working with ARTHUR BRUCKNER (1877–1975) at Basel, wrote the important chapter on heredity in ophthalmology in *Kurzes Handbuch der Ophthalmologie*, edited by F. Schieck of Würzburg and Bruckner.

1930   HARRY FRIEDENWALD (1864–1950) of Baltimore delivered the Doyne Lecture of the Oxford Ophthalmological Congress on 'The changes in the retinal vessels observed in arteriosclerosis and hypertension.'

1931   FRANCIS HEED ADLER (1895–1987) at the University of Pennsylvania published *Clinical physiology of the eye*, the first significant English text on ophthalmic physiology.

1931   JULES GONIN of Lausanne reported on his first series of 221 eyes in which the retinal break was localized and closed by perforating thermocauterization, his 'ignipuncture technique.' He reported a success rate of 53% with his technique.

1931   HOWARD CHRISTIAN NAFFZIGER (1884–1961) achieved decompression of the orbit by using the transfrontal approach for removal of the orbital wall.

1931   DAVID KARL LINDNER (1883–1961) and G. GUIST independently described their techniques for repairing retinal breaks to achieve chemical cauterization of the choroid using potassium hydroxide.

1931   While a research fellow at the Mayo Clinic, RAMON CASTROVIEJO (1904–1987) performed pioneering animal studies on corneal transplantation and published his findings in the *Proceedings of the Staff Meetings of the Mayo Clinic*.

1932   The second and definitive edition of WHITNALL's *The anatomy of the human orbit* appeared. This text still has utility today.

1932   FREDERICK H. VERHOEFF was appointed director of the Howe Laboratory. The location of the laboratory was moved from Harvard Medical School to the Massachusetts Eye and Ear Infirmary.

1932   SIR W. STEWART DUKE-ELDER published the first volume of his seven-volume *Textbook of ophthalmology*, completed in 1954. In the same year Duke-Elder operated on Ramsay McDonald, prime minister of England, for glaucoma.

1932   P. J. WAARDENBURG (1886–1979) in Leiden published *Das menschlichen Auge und seine Erbanlangen* (The human eye and its genetic disorders) that discussed familial eye diseases and presented an extensive collection of pedigrees. This work, together with the publication of JULES FRANÇOIS (1907–1984) in Ghent and FRONANCESCHETTI in Basel stimulated interest in ocular genetics.

1932   EDGAR DOUGLAS ADRIAN at Cambridge was awarded a Nobel Prize for work in electrophysiology that included a demonstration of electrical currents in the optic nerve, showing them to be a series of brief, frequent charges in potential. He shared the prize with SIR CHARLES SCOTT SHERRINGTON, who also contributed significantly to ophthalmic physiology.

1932   JOSEPH IMRE JR. of Budapest reintroduced the use of electrolysis in retinal reattachment surgery. AUREL VON SZILY and MACHEMER followed Imre with their use of both unipolar and bipolar electrolysis the following year.

1932   J. L. LACARRÈRE introduced diathermocoagulation, making use of a needle with two prongs, for applying traction to the lens in intracapsular lens extraction.

1932   SANFORD ROBINSON GIFFORD (1892–1945) of Omaha published *Handbook of ocular therapeutics*.

1933   T. J. DIMITRY modified the technique involved in phacoeresis (lens extraction with a suction cup) by using a syringe for suction.

1933   GIAMBATTISTA B. BIETTI (1907–1977) of Rome reported using cryotherapy to treat retinal tears. His method involved the use of carbon dioxide snow to produce a cryo-scar.

1933 EUGENE WOLFF (1896–1954), a London ophthalmologist and ophthalmic pathologist, published *The anatomy of the eye and orbit*. This became the standard anatomy text for ophthalmologists for more than half a century.

1933 ALAN CHURCHILL WOODS (1889–1963) of the Wilmer Institute published *Allergy and immunity in ophthalmology*, which stressed the roles of tuberculosis and focal infections in ocular inflammation.

1933 M. STEPHEN MAYOU of London modified the ophthalmoscope by introducing red-free light. This illumination made it less problematic to distinguish between pigment and blood in the fundus oculi.

1934 CLIFFORD B. WALKER (1884–1944) at Los Angeles described a modified method of applying diathermy in retinal detachment surgery that used 50% platinum–iridium wire.

1934 VLADIMIR PETROVICH FILATOV in Odessa demonstrated the utility of cadaver donor tissue in corneal transplant.

1934 JULES GONIN of Lausanne published his seminal work *Le décollement de la rétine* based on his experience with 38,000 patients and his lifelong study of the cause and treatment of retinal detachment.

1934 DIAZ-CANEJA introduced the use of infrared light in fundus photography, which allowed him to document choroidal circulation in the living eye.

1934 WILLIAM H. WILMER (1863–1936), the chair of ophthalmology at Johns Hopkins University, published *Atlas of the ocular fundus*, one of the most beautiful fundus atlases produced in the United States.

1934 G. H. STINE (1898–1952) developed a method to determine the precise localization of retinal breaks using a group of tables. The tables correlated the location of the retinal break with a location on the scleral surface.

1935 VLADIMIR PETROVICH FILATOV of Odessa published an article in *Archives of Ophthalmology* that recommended using corneas from enucleated eyes, refrigerated cadavers, and autoplastic material for use in corneal transplants.

1936 The Rohm and Haas Company introduced methyl methacrylate into the United States. This material replaced glass in many optical applications, as it was easier to mold and work than glass.

1936 CONRAD BERENS (1889–1963) of New York published *The eye and its diseases* to which 92 international authorities contributed.

1936   OTTO BARKAN of San Francisco published 'On the genesis of glaucoma,' a paper that used gonioscopy to categorize glaucoma. He also introduced techniques that made gonioscopy a routine diagnostic method for recognizing the feature of the angle-closure mechanism in the living eye.

1936   E. C. SEWELL introduced a technique for orbital decompression achieved by removing the medial wall of the orbit, allowing the orbital contents access to the ethmoid sinus.

1937   A. EDWARD DAVIS published *Medical treatment of cataracts*, in which he reported his study of lens antigen therapy, a nonsurgical treatment, to delay the advancement of cataracts. He reported that this treatment delayed the progress of the ordinary senile cataracts in up to 80% of cases when therapy was instituted early.

1937   DAME IDA CAROLINE MANN published her classic *Developmental abnormalities of the eye* which like her earlier *Development of the human eye* (1928) was drawn from the collection of human embryos of her mentor, W. ERNEST FRAZER of the University of London.

1937   GEORGE WALD (1906–1997), a professor of biology at Harvard, reported on the visual pigments, which he divided into two main types based on their absorption qualities. He retained the term 'rhodopsin' for the mammalian pigment (visual purple) and suggested 'poryphyropsin' for visual violet.

1937   L. MAMOLI described a technique for intraocular diathermy in which he introduced a diathermy needle thought the pars plana and applied transvitreal coagulation to posterior retinal breaks.

1937   Plastic (celluloid) contact lenses were developed by TEISSLER in Czechoslovakia.

1937   A. JESS was the first to describe the use of indentation or buckling of the sclera in retinal detachment surgery.

1937   CHARLES A. PERERA of New York presented, to the American Academy of Ophthalmology and Otolaryngology, his paper in which he proposed a classification of epithelium in the anterior chamber of the eye after operation and injury.

1937   HAROLD GLENDON SCHEIE (1909–1990) and G. D. GAMMON of Philadelphia reported the use of protigmin as a diagnostic test of myasthenia gravis.

1938   DAVID G. COGAN (1908–1993) at Harvard, in collaboration with R. LINDSAY REA of England, published *Neuro-ophthalmology*, a compilation of Cogan's neuro-ophthalmology lectures. This was the first book on the subject to have the word 'neuro-ophthalmology' in its title.

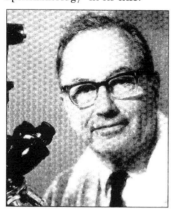

David Glendenning Cogan (1908–1993)
Courtesy of Francis A. Countway Library of Medicine,
Boston, MA.

1938　THEODOR E. OBRIG and F. MÜLLER independently introduced clear plastic scleral contact lenses in the United States. GYÖRFFY began fitting Plexiglas contact lenses.

1938　HANS GOLDMANN (1899–1991) of Zurich devised a contact lens to be used in conjunction with a slit lamp for viewing the angle of the anterior chamber.

1938　The Army Medical Museum issued an atlas consisting of photomicrographs of the eye in collaboration with and funded by the American Academy of Ophthalmology and Otolaryngology. These were used in the Academy's home study courses and in courses offered by the Army Medical Museum.

1938　DOHRMANN K. PISCHEL of San Francisco carried out the first scleral resection in the United States. He sometimes employed prior diathermy retinopexy and resected the sclera over areas of rigid retina.

1938　B. ROSENGREN at the Karolinska reported the use of an air bubble (gas tamponade) for temporary closure of retinal breaks.

1938　SANFORD ROBINSON GIFFORD published *Text-book of ophthalmology*. After Gifford's death, this book was continued by Adler, Scheie, and Albert.

1938　MORRIS B. BENDER (1905–1938), a neurologist from New York, collaborated with EDWINA WEINSTEIN to reveal the anatomy of internuclear ophthalmoplegia. Bender went on to study visual loss associated with cerebral lesions (1950s), optokinetic nystagmus (1950s), and the vestibular-ocular link (1960s).

1939　TUTOMU SATO (1902–1960) of Tokyo began his innovative studies on incisional refractive surgery. His long-term results in humans were disastrous because the important physiological role of the corneal endothelium was not yet recognized.

1939   BAYARD T. HORTON, ALEXANDER R. MACLEAN, and WINCHELL M. CRAIG at the Mayo Clinic published their description of cluster headaches, also known as histamine cephalalgia or Horton's headache in the *Proceedings of the Staff Meetings of the Mayo Clinic.*

1939   *The collected papers of John Martin Wheeler, M.D. on ophthalmic subjects* was published by his staff in the year following his death and was a valuable reference book for the field of ophthalmic plastic surgery for some years.

1939   EDMUND BENJAMIN SPAETH of Philadelphia published *Principles and practice of ophthalmic surgery.* The textbook became the model for oculoplastic texts.

1939   EARL CALVIN PADGETT (1893–1946) at the University of Kansas introduced the drum dermatome, providing an alternative to free full-thickness skin grafts.

1939   OTTO BARKAN of San Francisco introduced goniostomy as an operation in congenital glaucoma, believing this opened a membrane (Barkan's membrane) that prevented aqueous from reaching Schlemm's canal.

1940   HAROLD G. SCHEIE of Philadelphia reported on the site of disturbance in Adie's syndrome.

1940   FREDERICK ALLISON DAVIS (1883–1970), founder of the ophthalmology department at the University of Wisconsin – Madison, published a paper on primary tumors of the optic nerve, establishing the relationship between gliomas of the optic nerve and von Recklinghausen's disease.

1940   DAME IDA CAROLINE MANN and DAVIDINE PULLINGER of London reported on the pathology and improved treatment of mustard gas keratitis.

1940   The American Academy of Ophthalmology and Otolaryngology, under the direction of HARRY SEARLS GRADLE of Chicago, offered their first home study courses. These were eight correspondence courses directed toward ophthalmology resident training and were limited to basic sciences. The current ten-volume work *Basic and clinical science course* grew from this course. The set was published every year, and each volume covered an individual subspecialty.

1940   The first Pan-American Congress of Ophthalmology was held in Cleveland with HARRY SEARLS GRADLE as its president. Gradle served in this position until 1946.

1940	ALFRED BIELSCHOWSKY at the Dartmouth Eye Institute published *Lectures on motor anomalies*. Bielschowsky described his studies of ocular movement and his refined methods of afterimage observation technique by utilizing the perimeter.
1941	The Australian ophthalmologist NORMAN MCALISTER GREGG published his now-classic report on an epidemic of congenital cataracts and other ocular and cardiac problems linked to maternal infection with rubella virus during the first trimester.
1941	STEPHEN L. POLYAK of Chicago published *The retina: the anatomy and histology of the retina in man, ape and monkey*. It is a classic elucidation of the light microscopic structure of the retina as revealed by the Golgi technique.
1941	At the 1941 American Academy of Ophthalmology and Otolaryngology meeting, LUTHER C. PETER advocated the use of a mattress suture proposed earlier by Stallard for the closure of cataract incisions.
1941	FREDERICK MOHS at the University of Wisconsin – Madison described his technique of chemosurgery, allowing for a controlled method of cancer excision. This allowed for conservation of tissue and increased the cure rate for squamous cell carcinomas, basal cell carcinomas, and other skin tumors.
1941	KARL W. ASCHER (1887–1971) of Cincinnati discovered the aqueous veins and recognized their role in the circulation of the aqueous humor.
1942	THEODORE L. TERRY of Boston published the first histological description of retrolental fibroplasias, now known as retinopathy of prematurity.
1942	THEODOR E. OBRIG published *Contact lenses*, which detailed the development of contact lenses.
1942	Howard University appointed EDWIN J. WATSON as the chair of the ophthalmology department, the first African-American to head this department.
1943	WENDELL L. HUGHES (1900–1994), pupil of John Martin Wheeler, published *Reconstructive surgery of the eyelids*. Included in this excellent text is a wealth of historical detail.
1943	MILTON L. BERLINER of New York published *Biomicroscopy of the eye*, which included methods and outstanding illustrations. Berliner also provided a historical review of the slit-lamp biomicroscope.
1944	CHARLES WILBUR RUCKER of the Mayo Clinic published a description of venous sheathing in multiple sclerosis in the *Proceedings of the Staff*

Meetings of the Mayo Clinic.

1944   DOHRMANN K. PISCHEL developed an improved technique for applying diathermy in retinal detachment surgery using pins that were 20% platinum–iridium wire.

1944   R. TOWNLEY PATON of the Manhattan Eye, Ear, Nose, and Throat Hospital established the first eye bank to provide tissue for corneal transplants. It was located in New York City and was called the Eye Bank for Sight Restoration.

1944   W. R. HUGHES JR. and W. C. OWENS introduced their case study on cataract surgery at the American Academy of Ophthalmology and Otolaryngology. Drawing upon 3086 cases at the Wilmer Institute from 1925 to 1943, the findings supported the popular movement toward round pupil intracapsular surgery with corneoscleral sutures. The study showed that this method resulted in a decrease in the incidence of iris prolapse, hyphema, iridocyclitis, secondary glaucoma, retinal detachment, and postoperative astigmatism compared to other methods.

1944   JOHN MARQUIS CONVERSE (1909–1981) of New York described his technique for transnasal fixation of the medial canthal tendons in cases of traumatic telecanthus.

1944   RAYNOLD N. BERKE (1901–1986) presented his thesis 'Resection of the levator palpebrae for ptosis with anatomic studies,' to the American Ophthalmological Society. Berke, a faculty member at Columbia Presbyterian (1931) and later at Stanford University Medical School (1962), was a founding member of the American Society of Ophthalmic Plastic and Reconstructive Surgery (ASOPRS). He also collaborated with ALGERNON B. REESE to modify and reintroduce Krönlein's orbitotomy surgery.

1945   DAVID G. COGAN of Boston described the symptoms of nonsyphilitic interstitial keratitis, which came to be known as one of the 'Cogan syndromes.' The same year, Cogan published *The neurology of the ocular muscles.*

1945   CHARLES L. SCHEPENS (b. 1912) in Belgium designed the modern binocular indirect headband ophthalmoscope. Schepens's modifications were intended to facilitate the examination of retinal detachments. The initial instrument consisted of a headband that held the stereoscopic viewing system and a powerful light source fixed on a flexible, balanced arm. The examiner held a condensing lens in front of the patient's eye and saw an aerial image of the fundus.

1946   DAME IDA CAROLINE MANN demonstrated in rabbits the epithelial changes occurring in vitamin A deficiency.

1946	ALFRED KESTENBAUM, an American immigrant from Vienna who was on the staff at Bellevue, published *Clinical methods of neuro-ophthalmic examination*.
1946	ALBERT DARWIN RUEDEMANN SR. (1897–1971) of Cleveland, in an attempt to develop an implant with better motility following enucleation, developed an integrated plastic orbital consisting of a finished artificial eye anteriorly and a tantalum mesh posteriorly. The rectus muscles were attached to the mesh.
1946	NORMAN L. CUTLER developed a semiburied integrated ocular implant that had a ball and ring made of methyl methacrylate and had a square hole on its flat anterior surface. The artificial eye had a stem to fit into the hole.
1946	HERMENGILDO ARRUGA of Barcelona published *Cirugia ocular*. Arrugas's work was an important source of instruction for more than two decades.
1946	VLADIMIR PETROVICH FILATOV and VERBITSKA in Odessa published an article in the *American Review of Soviet Medicine* claiming successful results in 85 of 110 patients with retinitis pigmentosa treated with foreign protein therapy and the induction of sterile abscesses.
1946	KARL HRUBY in Vienna devised a precorneal concave lens that could be optically connected to a Haig-Streit slit lamp. This permitted examination of the vitreous cavity and fundus. This became known as the Hruby lens.
1946	HAROLD G. SCHEIE of Philadelphia and N. FREEMAN described the vascular disease associated with angioid streaks of the retina and pseudoxanthoma elasticum.
1947	FRANK BURTON WALSH (1895–1978) of Johns Hopkins, one of the founders of neuro-ophthalmology, published his monumental *Clinical neuro-ophthalmology*. It includes a synopsis of neuro-ophthalmic knowledge.
1947	MANUEL URIBE TRONCOSO (1868–1959) at the Harkness Eye Institute published *A treatise on gonioscopy*. This book is credited with elevating gonioscopy to an important clinical test. Troncoso also invented a monocular self-illuminating gonioscope.
1947	RICHARD G. SCOBEE (1914–1952) at Washington University published *The oculorotary muscles*. This was a synopsis of his 70 papers devoted to pediatric ophthalmology.
1947	HYLA BRISTOW STALLARD (1901–1973), a surgeon at Moorfields, modified Krönlein's lateral orbitotomy to obtain wider access to the orbit and to leave a more cosmetically satisfactory scar. His incision is

known as the Stallard–Wright technique.

1947   DAN M. GORDON, an ophthalmologist at Cornell Medical College, reported in the *American Journal of Ophthalmology* that in a study of 128 patients completing a course of Professor Filatov's foreign protein therapy he could not confirm Filatov's results.

1947   GEORGIANA DVORAK THEOBOLD of Chicago presented an important paper to the American Academy of Ophthalmology and Otolaryngology giving the first comprehensive histologic evidence of an association between delayed cataract wound healing and epithelial ingrowth.

1947   The American Academy of Ophthalmology and Otolaryngology sponsored the first conference on keratoplasty in Chicago. Ophthalmologists in the forefront of keratoplasty, such as R. TOWNLEY PATON, JOHN M. MCLEAN (1909–1968), RAMON CASTROVIEJO, and ALFRED EDWARD MAUMENEE, introduced their work in this area.

1947   The Ophthalmic Pathology Club, now known as the Verhoeff-Zimmerman Society, held its first meeting at the Army Institute of Pathology. The organization was founded by THEODORE SANDERS (St. Louis), JOHN MCLEAN (New York), and BENJAMIN RONES (Washington).

1948   J. B. BROWN and his colleagues improved Weiner's 1928 fascia lata sling procedure for ectropion by attaching the fascia to the frontalis and temporalis muscles.

1948   JONAS S. FRIEDENWALD and JACK S. GUYTON (1914–1987) of Baltimore revived frontalis muscle suspension for ptosis by using a permanent nonabsorbable suture. Their technique decreased the chance of late infections with the use of Supramid.

1948   HANS GOLDMANN in Zurich devised the three-mirror contact lens that provides improved stereoscopic visualization of the fundus.

1948   KEVIN TUOHY, an American optician, introduced an all-plastic

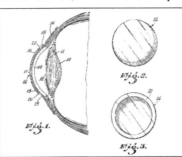

The Tuohy contact lens

corneal contact lens that was designed to float on top of a thin layer of tears covering the cornea.

1948   Z. TOTH suggested inserting a plastic canula after Critchett's three-snip procedure (1858), opening the canalicula in the treatment of epiphora.

1949   WALTER RUDOLF HESS (1881–1973), a Swiss ophthalmologist, was awarded the Nobel Prize for his studies on the physiology of the hypothalamus.

1949   JOHN S. MCGAVIC of Philadelphia described his technique for recurrent pterygia. He removed the entire pterygium and a significant amount of adjacent limbal conjunctiva and sutured the edge of the conjunctiva to the sclera. Postoperatively, he used beta-irradiation to control vascularization.

1949   RICHARD C. TROUTMAN (b. 1922) in New York introduced his buried, integrated magnetic ocular implant. Although clever in design, the implant caused significant conjunctival erosion due to its frequent slippage.

1949   GERD MEYER-SCHWICKERATH (1921–1992) of Germany initiated experiments with a high-intensity carbon arc lamp intended to produce clinical photocoagulation.

1949   JONAS S. FRIEDENWALD of Johns Hopkins gave the Jackson Memorial Lecture at the American Academy of Ophthalmology and Otolaryngology entitled 'A new approach to some problems of retinal vascular disease.' This classic lecture contained many of the contributions Friedenwald made on the pathogenesis of diabetic retinopathy, retrolental fibroplasias, and retinal arteriosclerosis.

1949   HAROLD RIDLEY of London performed the first intraocular lens implant after observing that certain plastics could be tolerated by ocular tissue. This occurred on November 29, and is one of the most important events in the history of cataract surgery.

1949   CYRIL DEE SHAPLAND at Moorfields devised a lamellar scleral resection procedure as an alternative to the older full-thickness scleral resection in the treatment of retinal detachment. Paufique, Huggonnier, and Dellaporta subsequently described similar scleral resection methods.

1949   HENRICUS JACOBUS MARIA WEVE of Utrecht developed a 'reefing' procedure for scleral shortening that consisted of taking lamellar suture bites in full-thickness sclera using a cross-stitch technique.

1949   HAROLD G. SCHEIE and B. JEROME of Philadelphia reported their technique for scleral shortening in retinal detachment surgery by brushing the surface of the sclera with a diathermy electrode. In the same year, Scheie described his favorable results using goniotomy in the treatment of congenital glaucoma.

1949   ERNST CUSTODIS (1898–1990) in Germany gave the first report of closing a retinal break by scleral buckling. Using compression sutures, he placed a polyvinyl cylinder on the sclera, which pushed the choroids against the retina.

1949   PHILIP SHOWALTER HENCH and his associates at the Mayo Clinic announced the alleviation of symptoms in rheumatoid arthritis patients treated with cortisone. The use of cortisone and related compounds soon proved useful in patients with certain inflammatory eye diseases.

1949   LEONARD CHRISTENSEN and KENNETH CARL SWAN (b. 1912) of Portland, Oregon, published their findings on the use of adrenergic blocking agents in the treatment of glaucoma.

1950   HELENOR CAMPBELL WILDER FOERSTER, working at the Armed Forces Institute of Pathology, first documented histopathologically nematode infections in the eye.

1950   HERBERT JAMES AMBROSE DARTNALL (b. 1914) at the Institute of Ophthalmology in London expanded and refined Wald's theories on cone and rod pigments. Between 1950 and 1959 he published his work based on his technique of partial bleaching, finding that there were more than the two rod pigments (rhodopsin and porphyropsin) proposed by Wald.

1950   ALSTON CALLAHAN (b. 1911) in Birmingham, Alabama published *Surgery of the eye—injuries*. This was based upon his experience in World War II.

1950   HYLA BRISTOW STALLARD in London published *Eye surgery*.

1950   HANS GOLDMANN of Zurich developed his bowl perimeter that allowed for perimetric testing statically or kinetically.

1950   FRANCIS HEED ADLER of Philadelphia published *Physiology of the eye: clinical applications*. The same year, Adler was appointed editor-in-chief of the *Archives of Ophthalmology*.

1950   DANIEL B. KIRBY at Bellevue published *Surgery of cataract*. Published at the height of popularity for intracapsular cataract extraction, it highlighted the chronology of cataract surgery.

1950   WALTER MORTON GRANT (1915–2002) in the Howe Laboratory introduced tonography to detect abnormal resistance to outflow located within the outflow channels.

1950   OSKAR HIRSCH (b. 1877) described surgical decompression for malignant exophthalmos by removal of the orbital floor, allowing access to the maxillary sinus.

1950   HAROLD G. SCHEIE of Philadelphia described goniopuncture, a new filtering operation for the treatment of congenital glaucoma.

1951   A monograph by MICHAEL J. HOGAN of San Francisco on toxoplasmosis uveitis was published. This work is considered a classic in the field.

1951   SAVADORE CASTAÑARES improved the understanding of ocular anatomy with his description of the distinct fat compartments of the upper and lower orbit and their relations. He also emphasized the importance of the orbicularis muscle, including its hypertrophy and excision in regard to cosmetic blepharoplasty.

1951   SYDNEY A. FOX (1898–1983) of New York improved lower lid entropion with a modified triangular tarsal excision. This method, originally introduced by von Graefe in 1864, gained wide acceptance following Fox's publication.

1951   ALGERNON BEVERLY REESE (1896–1981) of New York published *Tumors of the eye*. This book was influential in both ocular oncology and ophthalmic pathology.

1951   CHARLES L. SCHEPENS improved his binocular indirect headband ophthalmoscope by incorporating the stereoscopic viewing system and a powerful light source into the headband. Schepens and his colleagues in the same year also performed the first scleral buckling procedures in the United States using foreign materials.

1951   E. M. JACK and A. B. KATZNELSON were the first to attempt to substitute saliva for tears by transplanting Stenson's duct into the lower fornix in patients with dry eyes.

1952   JONAS S. FRIEDENWALD'S text *The pathology of the eye* was expanded and merged with the *Atlas of ophthalmic pathology* by DE COURSEY and ASH. The new work was entitled *Ophthalmic pathology: an atlas and textbook*.

1952   JOHN MARQUIS CONVERSE and BYRON CAPLEESE SMITH (1908–1990) of New York introduced their orbital floor reconstruction surgery that made use of bone grafts.

1952   GEORGE M. HAIK of New Orleans and his colleagues reported on the application of beta-irradiation using a radium applicator following surgery for pterygium excision. This significantly reduced the rate of recurrence. They later changed their beta-irradiation applicator to a strontium-90 (1957).

1952   FREDERICK W. STOCKER at Duke University presented his work on corneal endothelium in keratoplasty. He showed that the corneal endothelium was vital for preserving corneal dehydration.

1952   A. BARON in France introduced anterior chamber lens implantation. The results, however, were less than satisfactory in the long run, resulting in corneal edema and glaucoma.

1952   SYDNEY FOX of New York introduced the term 'dermachalasis' (or 'dermatochalasis' as currently used) to describe the 'baggy eyelid deformity.' In the same year, Fox published *Ophthalmic plastic surgery*, in which he introduced his Z-plasty method for entropion surgery.

1952   HELENOR CAMPBELL WILDER FOERSTER at the Armed Forces Institute of Pathology first reported the finding of *Toxoplasma* organisms in necrotic retina in granulomatous chorioretinal lesions in 53 eyes that she studied.

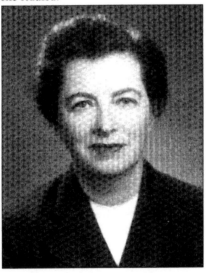

Helenor Campbell Wilder Foerster

1952   DAVID G. COGAN of Boston first reported 'Cogan's ocular motor apraxia.'

1952   DOHRMANN K. PISCHEL of San Francisco used the direct ophthalmoscope to pinpoint retinal breaks.

1952   LESTER T. JONES (1894–1983) advocated an endonasal approach for dacryocystorhinostomy.

1952   GERD MEYER-SCHWICKERATH in Germany began treating small melanomas and retinal angiomas with photocoagulation.

1952   ARNALL PATZ (b. 1920) of Baltimore and coworkers reported their studies in the newborn nursery linking high oxygen administration to retrolental fibroplasias.

1953   EDWARD EPSTEIN in South Africa performed the first intraocular lens implantation that used an iris-fixation lens or 'collar stud lens.' He later switched to a pupillary iris plane lens (Copeland lens).

1953   CHARLES E. ILIFF (b. 1911) of Johns Hopkins introduced a simplified ptosis procedure using the posterior approach in which he employed a clamp to shorten the posterior lamella. This further popularized the posterior approach.

1954   BERNARD BECKER (b. 1920) of St. Louis and WALTER MORTON GRANT in Boston introduced the use of Diamox (acetazolamide), a drug that lowers IOP through decreased aqueous humor production.

1954   RICHARD M. BURKE offered an additional modification of the Krönlein procedure surgery to gain more extensive access to the orbit and to leave a smaller scar.

1954   B. STRAMPELLI in Rome gave the initial description of retinal reattachment operations in which absorbable dried gelatin sponge was employed. This created temporary buckling that allowed for the formation of chorioretinal adhesions.

1954   HANS LITTMAN gave the first report of the modern operating microscope that consisted of a 'telecentric device with a constant working distance, a Galilean turret for changing magnification, and a paraxial illumination source.'

1954   VICTOR EVERETT KINSEY (1909–1978) and F. M. HEMPHILL published the preliminary report of the cooperative study of retrolental fibroplasia and incriminated oxygen as the cause.

1955   PAUL LOUIS TESSIER repopularized Borguet's transconjunctival approach to lower lid fat excision when he utilized it for attaining access to the orbital floor.

1955   NORMAN L. CUTLER in San Fancisco and CROWELL J. BEARD (b. 1912) introduced their upper eyelid reconstruction method consisting of a temporary blepharorrhaphy by means of a pedicle of full-thickness lower eyelid advanced beneath a bridge of the lower eyelid margin, now referred to as the Cutler–Beard bridge-flap.

1955   HANS GOLDMANN at Bern introduced his applanation tonometer, which avoids the artifacts of the Schiotz tonometer and remains the most reliable method of estimating intraocular pressure.

1955   EVERETT R. VEIRS (b. 1908) of Temple, Texas published *The lacrimal system, clinical application*.

1955   GERD MEYER-SCHWICKERATH introduced the use of photocoagulation for treating diabetic retinopathy.

1955   B. STRAMPELLI in Rome introduced anterior chamber implants.

1955   VLADIMIR PETROVICH FILATOV in Odessa reported on his series of 3500 corneal transplants done with a success rate of 60% to 65% and in selected cases up to 90%.

1955   WILLIAM G. EVERETT of Pittsburg devised an 'outfolding' method for scleral shortening surgery in the treatment of retinal detachment. It involved a full-thickness radial scleral incision with circumferential undermining to create a mobile band of sclera. Mattress sutures through the zone of mobile sclera when tightened resulted in outward folding of the sclera.

1955   FREDERICK CARL CORDES (1892–1965) of San Francisco presented, to the American Academy of Ophthalmology and Otolaryngology, his work on congenital cataract surgery procedures. Cordes recommended that, in terms of immediate results and decreased complications, linear extraction was the safest. Multiple needles seemed to Cordes to be the least desirable of all procedures.

1955   ARNALL PATZ began his important work at the Wilmer Institute on retinopathy of prematurity and diabetic retinopathy.

1955   HAROLD G. SCHEIE and MELVIN G. ALPER (b. 1921) at the University of Pennsylvania described the treatment of herpes zoster ophthalmicus with cortisone and corticotropin.

1956   The Zeiss optical microscope was adapted for ocular surgery by H. HARMS (b. 1908) in Tübingen and JOAQUIN BARRAQUER in Barcelona. This method rapidly became standard for intraocular surgery.

1956   FRANÇOIS HERVOUËT and PAUL LOUIS TESSIER of France proposed a combined posterior tarsectomy with an anterior resection of skin and muscle for the correction of ptosis.

1956   G. HENRY MUNDT JR. and WILLIAM FRANKLIN HUGHES JR. were the first to demonstrate the usefulness of ultrasound technology in ophthalmology.

1956   PETER CHOYCE introduced the first practical anterior chamber implant, which he modified nine times during the next 13 years.

1956–1961   ALAN CHURCHILL WOODS of the Wilmer Institute published a book of his work on ocular inflammations, *Endogenous uveitis*.

1956   MAX CHAMLIN at Einstein Medical Center and K. RUBNER reported a method of retinal detachment repair in which two parallel areas of lamellar dissection were combined to enhance the buckling effect.

1956   BOBERG-ANS improved Frey's original method to test corneal sensitivity by means of a series of hairs. Boberg-Ans substituted for the hairs nylon threads that were better suited for the measurement of pressure. He also introduced the use of focused air currents directed at the eye.

1956   GERD MEYER-SCHWICKERATH in Germany developed a xenon arc photocoagulator in cooperation with Hans Littman and the Zeiss Optical Company.

1956   E. H. LAMBERT, L. M. EATON, and E. D. ROOKE of the Mayo Clinic published in the *American Journal of Physiology* the association of a defect in neuromuscular transmission and malignancy (Lambert–Eaton syndrome).

1956   JOHN WARREN HENDERSON (b. 1912) of the Mayo Clinic published his thesis on essential blepharospasm.

1957   OTTO LOWENSTEIN at the Harkness Eye Institute constructed a direct-writing infrared electronic pupillograph.

1957   CORNELIUS D. BINKHORST at Sluiskill in the Netherlands developed his iris-clip lens.

1957   BYRON CAPLEESE SMITH, a student of WENDELL HUGHES, and WILLIAM REGAN, Smith's resident, coined the term 'blowout fractures' for orbital floor fractures.

1957   SAUL H. SUGAR (1912–1993), head of Detroit's Sinai Hospital Department of Ophthalmology and professor and chief of the glaucoma service at Wayne State University Medical School, published *The glaucomas*.

1957   The Gonin Medal, in honor of JULES GONIN, was established by the University of Lausanne and the Swiss Ophthalmological Society. Past recipients include Hermenegildo Arruga and Gerd Meyer-Schwickerath, and Alan Churchill Woods of Baltimore.

1957   THEODORE E. WALSH and JOSEPH H. OGURA (b. 1915) introduced their Caldwell–Luc approach for removal of the floor and medial wall of the orbit.

1957   A team of Chinese researchers in Peking, headed by TIANG, was the first to isolate and culture *Chlamydia trachomatis*, the etiologic agent of trachoma.

1957   MATTHEW ALPERN used the entoptic perception of the observer's fovea in the study of ocular movements.

1957   DUPONT GUERRY and his colleagues performed the first successful photocoagulation therapy in the United States using a carbon arc searchlight as a light source. They treated a retinal hemangioma.

1957	JOAQUIN BARRAQUER of Barcelona introduced alphachymotrypsin in cataract extraction.
1957	DAVID D. DONALDSON of Harvard, in conjunction with HAROLD EDGERTON of the Massachusetts Institute of Technology, designed a retinal camera that took simultaneous stereoscopic photographs utilizing an electronic flash tube with a duration of 1/1000 second.
1957	BENJAMIN RONES and LORENZ E. ZIMMERMAN of Washington report the production of heterochromia glaucoma by diffuse malignant melanoma of the iris.
1958	*The vertebrate visual system*, by STEPHEN L. POLYAK, was published posthumously. It included a compilation of neuro-anatomy literature of the eye, the brain, and the 'visual pathway.'
1958	SIR W. STEWART DUKE-ELDER published the first of his 15-volume *System of ophthalmology*, the last volume was published in 1976.
1958	DANIEL VAUGHN and TAYLOR ASBURY published *General ophthalmology*. The book was meant for general medicine specialists.
1958	JULES FRANÇOIS of Ghent published his important text on ophthalmic genetics entitled *L'hérédité en ophtalmologie*. The following year, François published *Les cataractes congénitales* (1959).
1958	R. A. PERRITT was among the first to describe microsurgery of the eye; he used a stable binocular microscope.
1958	G. CLARK, who was among the first to recommend lamellar scleral flaps for routine scleral buckling, described a technique for lamellar dissection preserving the scleral flap.
1958	JOAQUIN BARRAQUER of Barcelona reported the use of a–chymotrypsin for enzymatic zonulolysis in facilitating intracapsular cataract extraction. This was a major advance over breaking the zonules with an instrument.
1958	ALBERT N. LEMOINE of Kansas City, Missouri, and his colleagues reported on a scleral imbrication method in which the buckling effect was placed to support the retinal break on its anterior slope.
1958	HERMENEGILDO ARRUGA of Barcelona reported nonabsorbable sutures used for ringing the globe during scleral buckling surgery. While popular in Europe, this procedure was often complicated by rapid transscleral erosion of the suture.
1958	CHARLES H. TOWNES of Columbia University and A. L. SCHAWLOW proposed the modern laser instrument, which emitted powerful, coherent visible monochromatic wavelengths.
1958	HAROLD G. SCHEIE of Philadelphia utilized scleral cautery to produce

retraction of scleral wound edges in a fistulizing procedure for the treatment of glaucoma (Scheie procedure).

1958   LORENZ E. ZIMMERMAN and F. B. JOHNSON demonstrated oxylate crystals within ocular tissues.

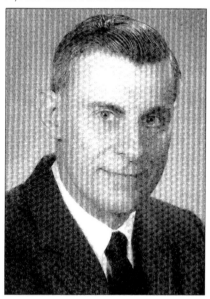

Lorenz E. Zimmerman

1958   THOMAS P. KEARNS (b. 1922) of the Mayo Clinic, in collaboration with pathologist GEORGE P. SAYRE, published in the *Archives of Ophthalmology* a report of two patients with retinitis pigmentosa, external ophthalmoplegia, and cardiomyopathy (Kearns–Sayre syndrome).

1959   KENNETH CARL SWAN described his method for scleral imbrication, in which the buckling was attained by mattress sutures that folded the anterior scleral flap under the posterior flap.

1959   V. CAVKA, professor at Belgrade, introduced an alternative method for scleral imbrication in which the buckling was attained through a scleral flap.

1959   GERD MEYER-SCHWICKERATH published *Lichtkoagulation*, summarizing the use of photocoagulation and laser treatment up to that time.

1959   MACKENSEN and HARMS at Tübingen began using Perlon (nylon) sutures in intraocular surgery.

1959   MILTON FLOCKS and coworkers at Stanford investigated the retinal circulation in cats using various injectable dyes and cinephotography.

1959   BENJAMIN RONES and LORENZ E. ZIMMERMAN demonstrated the excellent prognosis of iris melanomas treated by iridectomy.

1959   BEN S. FINE and coworkers in Washington published 'Some general principles of electron microscopy,' helping to establish the importance of electron microscopy in ophthalmic pathology.

1960   LORENZ E. ZIMMERMAN of the Armed Forces Institute of Pathology elucidated the nature of melanocytomas in his De Schweinitz lecture, 'Pigmented tumors of the optic nerve head.'

1960   PAUL AUSTIN CHANDLER (1896–1987) of Boston and A. EDWARD MAUMENEE (1913–1998) of Baltimore presented evidence that the cause hypotony following cataract surgery in the absence of external filtration is a serous detachment of the ciliary body.

1960   THEODORE HAROLD MAIMAN built the first functional medical laser using a pink ruby as the active material.

1960   CHARLES L. SCHEPENS and his colleagues in Boston refined their scleral buckling technique with the addition of silicone rubber implants.

1960   H. R. NOVOTNY and D. L. ALVIS introduced photographic angiography of the retinal circulation using sodium fluorescein as a dye. This technique has become an invaluable diagnostic tool.

1960   HARVEY E. THORPE (d. 1982) of Pittsburgh gave the initial report of scleral buckling operations that made use of autologous fascia lata from the thigh.

1960   A. L. MACLEAN and A. EDWARD MAUMENEE of Baltimore carried out angioscopy by injecting fluorescein intravenously into patients with choroidal tumors during ophthalmoscopic examination.

1960   JULES STEIN, an ophthalmologist who served his residency at Cook County Hospital, founded the Research to Prevent Blindness foundation for the advancement of eye research.

1960   LORENZ E. ZIMMERMAN and BRADLEY R. STRAATSMA (b. 1927) at the Armed Forces Institute of Pathology reported on the anatomical relationships of the retina to the vitreous body and to the pigment epithelium.

1961   ROBERT W. HOLLENHORST (b. 1913) of the Mayo Clinic described in JAMA cholesterol plaques in the retinal circulation as a sign of cartid occlusive disease (Hollenhorst plaques).

1961   LESTER T. JONES of Portland, Oregon, described his technique of managing canalicular obstruction with conjuctivorhinostomy using Pyrex tubes to provide a pathway between the lacrimal lake and the nose. Jones emphasized an anatomical approach to problems of the

214

eyelids and lacrimal apparatus.

1961   ROCKO M. FASANELLA, chairman of the Department of Ophthalmology at Yale, and JAVIER SERVAT (d. 2000), Fasanella's resident, introduced their tarsectomy surgery that resected Müller's muscle for minimum ptosis correction. This became known as the Fasanella–Servat procedure.

1961   MILTON M. ZARET and coworkers published their work on the effects of ruby laser photocoagulation in animals.

1961   MARY F. LYON published evidence for X-linked human disease using ocular albinism as an illustration.

1961   DAVID KASNER (b. 1927) of Miami began the practice of partial anterior vitrectomy in the intraoperative management of vitreous loss in cataract surgery. This was first done using sponges and later with automated vitreatomy devices.

1961   The Eye Bank Association of America was founded. Their data indicated that approximately 2000 corneal transplants were performed in the United States that year.

1961   BERNARD BECKER of St. Louis and ROBERT N. SHAFFER published *Diagnosis and therapy of the glaucomas*. This text brought together current thinking concerning the pathogenesis, diagnosis, and management of the glaucomas and helped to popularize gonioscopy.

1961   KARL W. ASCHER of Cincinnati published *The aqeous veins*. This brought to the attention of ophthalmologists his groundbreaking work on the circulation of the aqueous humor, i.e. the aqueous veins.

1961   WENDELL L. HUGHES of New York supervised the writing of *Ophthalmic plastic surgery* for the American Academy of Ophthalmology and Otolaryngology.

1961   The Hans Littmann diploscope was introduced. It consisted of two surgical microscopes attached to one another with common paths for illumination and observation achieved through a system of prisms. This was a major advance in surgical teaching.

1961   WALLACE S. FOULDS of Glasgow was the first to recommend a preliminary trial of canalicular closure in patients with dry eyes. He inserted gelatin rods into the canaliculi.

1961   T. KRWAWICZ of Lublin, Poland, pioneered cryoextraction for intracapsular cataract surgery. Cryoextraction proved easier and more secure than previous forceps or suction methods.

1961   A. BORRÁS introduced the use of gelatin as a resorbable intrascleral implant.

215

1961	H. A. MILLER and M. LAROCHE of France used preserved human sclera as a buckling material in retinal detachment surgery.
1961	HOWARD NAQUIN and SIR BENJAMIN RYCROFT (1902–1967) the following year published their updated techniques for Collies's 1864 exenteration operation.
1962	MICHAEL J. HOGAN and LORENZ ZIMMERMAN coedited *Ophthalmic pathology: an atlas and textbook*.
1962	WALTER MORTON GRANT, a glaucoma specialist from Boston, published *Toxicology of the eye*, focusing on drugs with adverse ocular effects.
1962	The rubella virus was isolated and cultivated in tissue culture at the Harvard School of Public Health and at Walter Reed Army Institute of Research in Washington, D.C.
1962	CHARLES D. KELMAN (b. 1930) in New York City developed the first hand-held cryostylet for cataract removal.
1962	CHARLES D. J. REGAN and associates in Boston used a silicone band in retinal detachment surgery in place of the polyethylene tube. This lessened the risk of transscleral erosion and removed the 'dead space' in the lumen of the tube, which decreased the chance of infection.
1962	CLAES H. DOHLMAN (b. 1922) of Boston and coworkers reported on the swelling pressure of the corneal stroma. This was followed by Dohlman's additional important studies regarding fluid physiology and nutrition of the cornea.
1962	LOUIS J. GIRARD and ALICE R. MCPHERSON (b. 1926) reported an innovative technique of scleral buckling in retinal detachment surgery. This was a full thickness and circumferential technique using a solid silicone rubber rod.
1962	SIR BENJAMIN WILLIAM RYCROFT, author of the first book in English on keratoplasty, played a major role in the passage of the Human Tissue Act.
1962	DAVID KASNER of Miami developed the concept of planned open-sky vitrectomy with his operation that deliberately removed the vitreous gel, initially with cellulose sponges and scissors.
1962	F. RODRIGUEZ-VASQUEZ gave the initial report on the use of preserved human sclera in buckling operations in the American literature.
1962	In this and the following year, THOMAS D. DUANE (1917–1993) of Philadelphia, in a study commissioned by Research to Prevent Blindness, published *Ophthalmic research U.S.A.* This study concluded that there was a need for a National Eye Institute to deal

with the problem of 30,000 new blind patients each year in the United States.

1962   EVERETT R. VEIRS in Temple, Texas, described the use of malleable metal rods (Veirs rods) in the repair of traumatically severed lacrimal canaliculi.

1962   HAROLD G. SCHEIE, GEORGE W. HAMBRICK and LOUIS A. BARNES describe a 'forme fruste' of Hurler's disease (Scheie's syndrome).

1962   J. F. PORTERFIELD and LORENZ E. ZIMMERMAN at the Armed Forces Institute of Pathology published their classic article on rhabdomyosarcoma of the orbit.

1963   HERBERT E. KAUFMAN (b. 1931), E. L. MARTOLA, and CLAES H. DOHLMAN in Boston report the successful treatment of herpes simplex infection of the cornea with 5-Iodo-2-deoxyuridine (IDU, IDUR), an antiviral drug developed by WILLIAM H. PRUSOFF at Yale.

1963   Using linkage analysis, J. H. RENWICK and S. D. LAWLER demonstated probable linkage between a congenital cataract locus and the Duffy blood group locus.

1963   RICHARD C. TROUTMAN introduced the use of nylon sutures and microscopic surgery for keratoplasty in the United States.

1963   N. KUNITOMO and S. MORI of Japan introduced the application of mitomycin for the treatment of pterygia. In subsequent studies by SINGH and his colleagues, it was found that the rate of recurrence was greatly reduced with the mitomycin therapy.

1963   CHARLES J. CAMPBELL and his associates in New York City and MILTON FLOCKS and his associates in Palo Alto independently reported the effects of ruby laser photocoagulation in human eyes.

1963   HELENA BIANTOVSKAVA FEDUKOWICZ (1900–1998) of New York University published the first book in the English language devoted entirely to ocular clinical bacteriology, *External infections of the eye: bacterial, viral and mycotic.*

1963   ADOLPHE FRANCESCHETTI of Geneva, JULES FRANÇOIS OF GHENT, and J. BABEL of France published *Les hérédo-dégénerescences chorio-rétiniennes.* This work was a significant contribution to the understanding of the heredity of eye diseases.

1963   CHARLES KELMAN and T. S. COOPER used Cooper-Linde's croptherapy instrument to produce a chorioretinal scar.

1963   H. NEUBAUER invented intravitreal scissors with hinged blades controlled by finger pressure.

1963   ROBERT H. FENTON (b. 1931) and LORENZ E. ZIMMERMAN at the

Armed Forces Institue of Pathology described hemolytic glaucoma, now often referred to as 'ghost cell glaucoma.'

1964   RAMON CASTROVIEJO of New York, a pioneer in corneal transplantation, published *Atlas de queratectomías y queratoplastias* that summarized his techniques and experience in keratoplasty.

1964   MORRIS B. BENDER of New York published *The oculomotor system*. This was the outcome of a symposium held at Mount Sinai Hospital on eye movement control.

1964   JOSÉ IGNACIO BARRAQUER (1916–1998) of Bogota, Colombia introduced his lamellar keratectomy surgery method of cryolathe keratomileusis.

1964   ALAN B. SCOTT (b. 1932) of San Francisco described scleral buckling methods that used plantaris tendon to encircle the globe.

1964   HARVEY LINCOFF and JOHN M. MCLEAN in New York City described their technique for cryosurgical treatment of retinal detachment.

1964   J. LAWTON SMITH (b. 1929) and JOEL S. GLASER (b. 1938) published the first volume of the *University of Miami neuro-ophthalmology symposia*.

1964   HARRY A. EASOM (b. 1933) and LORENZ E. ZIMMERMAN at the Armed Forces Institute of Pathology demonstrated the clinicopathologic correlation between sympathetic ophthalmica and bilateral phacoanaphylaxis.

1964   ANDREW P. FERRY (b. 1929) and LORENZ E. ZIMMERMAN At the Armed Forces Institute of Pathology described 'black cornea' as a complication of the topical use of epinephrine.

1964   The first report of an intracorneal plastic lens is published in the *Mayo Clinic Proceedings* by JOHN WARREN HENDERSON and PAUL G. BELAU of the Mayo Clinic.

1965   CROWELL J. BEARD of San Francisco introduced the use of bilateral fascia lata brow suspension with destruction of the normal levator muscle for the treatment of unilateral congenital ptosis and for ptosis with jaw-winking.

1965   GUNNAR B. STICKLER and colleagues at the Mayo Clinic describe a new syndrome, hereditary progressive arthro-ophthalmopathy in the *Mayo Clinic Proceedings*.

1965   PAUL LOUIS TESSIER presented the first case of modern craniofacial surgery at the meeting of the French Society of Plastic Surgery. He is widely regarded as the founder of the field of craniofacial surgery and was a leader in bone grafting methods.

1965   S. P. AMOILS reported on his cryoprobe, which was based on the Jule Thompson principle that rapid expansion of a compressed gas causes a drop in temperature. The Amoils cryoprobe could be adjusted to go as low as -70° C.

1965   PAUL A. CHANDLER and WALTER MORTON GRANT of the Massachusetts Eye and Ear Infirmary assembled and edited the series of outstanding lectures they gave on glaucoma into *Lectures on glaucoma*. They worded both research aspects and surgical techniques.

1965   CORNELIUS D. BINKHORST in the Netherlands designed a two-loop iridocapsular intraocular lens.

1965   The first motorized microscope appeared; the magnification was adjustable through a footpedal mechanism. This allowed the user to change magnification without interrupting the operation to make a manual adjustment.

1965   PAUL CIBIS (1911–1965) of St. Louis published *Vitreoretinal pathology and surgery in retinal detachments*. The same year Cibis invented an 'intravitreal tissue cutter' that involved the band being caught with a hook and cut by moving a trephine. He also gave the initial report of intraocular cryotherapy using an intravitreal cryoprobe and successfully treated retinal detachments with silicone oil.

1965   ROBERT BROCKHURST and coworkers in Boston suggested further modification in the lamellar scleral dissection method of scleral buckling together with staggered diathermy in the bed of the dissection and the use of intrascleral implants of various types. This became the 'classic' scleral buckling technique.

1965   HARVEY A. LINCOFF and his colleagues refined Custodis's episcleral exoplant method by substituting a silicone sponge for the polyviol exoplant, introducing an improved needle for placing scleral sutures, and subsequently replacing cryotherapy with diathermy.

1965   LORENZ E. ZIMMERMAN at the Armed Forces Institute of Pathology described in detail the ocular and orbital lesions of juvenile xanthogranuloma. In the same year he presented his study of the pathogenesis of rubella cataracts in Gregg's syndrome.

1966   MORTON E. SMITH (b. 1934) and coworkers at the Armed Forces Institute of Pathology described ocular involvement in congenital cytomegalic inclusion disease.

1966   FRANCIS A. L'ESPERANCE started research on producing an argon laser for clinical use.

1966   MALCOLM W. BICK repopularized von Ammon's full-thickness triangle ectropion operation (1831) with his technique for lateral resection of the eyelid.

1966   J. R. CASSADY, B. S. T. L. LIDDY, and G. A. JOSELSON independently suggested the use of thiotepa, a mustard nitrogen analog, as adjunctive therapy after pterygium excision to reduce the recurrence rate.

1966   WILLIAM FLETCHER HOYT, the distinguished San Francisco neuro-ophthalmologist, and DIANE BEESTON, a photographer, published *The ocular fundus in neurologic disease: a diagnostic manual and stereo atlas*.

1966   JOHN CLARK MUSTARDÉ published *Repair and reconstruction in the orbital region*. Two of his methods include the 'Mustardé flying man technique' and the 'Mustardé cheek flap,' both of which are still currently employed.

1966   ALSTON CALLAHAN published *Reconstructive surgery of the eyelids and ocular adnexa*. Callahan's book presented techniques of medial canthal fixation, composite lid grafting, and levator recession.

1966   DAVID D. DONALDSON of Boston published the first volume of his five-volume work, *Atlas of external diseases of the eye: Congenital anomalies and systemic diseases*. The final volume, *The crystalline lens*, was published in 1976.

1966   DAME IDA C. MANN, now at the Royal Perth Hospital in Australia, published *Culture, race, climate and eye diseases*, a culmination of her scientific observations and travel experiences.

1966   FRANCIS A. L'ESPERANCE introduced absorbable collagen as a material for use in scleral buckling.

1966   GOTTFRIED O. NAUMAN (b. 1935), MYRON YANOFF (b. 1936), and LORENZ E. ZIMMERMAN of the Armed Forces Institue of Pathology presented their histopathologic study linking the histogenesis of uveal melanomas to nevi.

1966   ROBERT MACHEMER (b. 1933) in Miami reported the first case of a patient with bilateral diffuse uveal melanocytic proliferation.

1967   J. DONALD M. GASS (b. 1928) of Miami published his classic monograph, *Pathogenesis of disciform detachment of the neuroepithelium*.

1967   V. ARATOON of Baghdad published the encouraging results of his pterygium procedure, which involved covering the pterygium excision site with a pedicle flap.

1967   GEORGE WALD and HALDAN KEFFER HARTLINE (1903–1983) received the Nobel Prize in physiology or medicine for their studies of the visual pigments and the discovery of simple retinal receptor responses. RAGNAR ARTHUR GRANIT (1900–1991) at the Karolinska

Institute also received the Nobel Prize for recording electrical impulses from single optic nerve fibers without dissection by using microelectrodes.

1967   H. MACKENZIE FREEMAN of Boston developed scissors activated by finger pressure, which were useful in cutting vitreous bonds by advancing a tubular shaft to close the blades.

1967   CHARLES D. KELMAN of New York devised the first apparatus for phacoemulsification, fragmenting soft lens material by ultrasound energy and then irrigating and aspirating it. This was a major advance in cataract surgery.

1967   ALICE R. MCPHERSON of Houston published her chapter on cryosurgery in the prophylaxis and management of retinal detachment in E. B. Streiff's *Modern problems in ophthalmology*.

1967   W. RICHARD GREEN and LORENZ E. ZIMMERMAN at the Armed Forces Institute of Pathology describe a granulomatous reaction to Descemet's membrane in herpes simplex infection.

1967   CLAES H. DOHLMAN and MIGUEL F. REFOJO of Boston and coworkers reported on the use of sympathetic polymers in corneal surgery.

1968   MARTIN H. VOGEL (b. 1935), RAMON L. FONT (b. 1930) and LORENZ E. ZIMMERMAN at the Armed Forces Institute of Pathology presented a detailed clinicopathologic description of six cases of 'reticulum cell sarcoma' (large cell lymphoma) of the retina and uvea.

1968   J. DONALD M. GASS published 'A fluorescein angiographic study of macular dysfunction secondary to retinal vascular disease: parts I to VI'. In the same year, Gass and E. W. D. NORTON presented evidence that cystoid macular edema following cataract extractions was caused by exudate from capillaries being soaked up by the Henle plexiform band.

1968   SIDNEY FOX of New York published the first major text devoted solely to eyelid ptosis surgery, *Surgery of ptosis*. Fox stressed the variety of ways ptosis could be improved.

1968   MOLTENO reported the use of a seton, composed of a plastic tube, for the treatment of glaucoma. The seton transports aqueous from the anterior chamber to an acrylic plate to a new drainage area behind the eye.

1968   DAVID MAURICE at Stanford developed the specular microscope. This instrument permitted the corneal endothelium to be studied.

1968   POMERANTZEFF in Boston applied Gullstrand's principle to the Schepens ophthalmoscope and produced an improved version that avoided reflections from the patient's cornea and crystalline lens. The

Schepens ophthalmoscope serves as the basis for the many models of indirect ophthalmoscopes used today.

1969   HERMENEGILDO ARRUGA in his last paper reported on his results of 1000 operations using a modified tube technique for the repair of retinal detachment.

1969   As a measure to study lens implantations, community ophthalmologists in the United States agreed to stop all lens implantations for two years to examine the 243 completed surgeries. The examinations revealed that the implants were sufficiently favorable to permit a continuance of lens implantation surgery.

1969   CROWELL BEARD of San Francisco published his classic *Ptosis*.

1969   A vaccine against rubella virus infection was licensed in the United States, effectively putting an end to rubella epidemics and the resultant congenital cataracts.

1969   FRANCIS A. L'ESPERANCE at Columbia reported argon laser treatment of a human eye. HUNTER L. LITTLE and his colleagues in Palo Alto also treated the patients with argon laser in the same year.

1969   MARK O. M. TSO (b. 1936), BEN S. FINE and LORENZ E. ZIMMERMAN at the Armed Forces Institute of Pathology described 'fluerettes' showing photoreceptor differentiation in retinoblastomas and with ROBERT M. ELLSWORTH (1928–1994) of New York documented the radioresistence to tumor with this feature.

1970   HUNTER L. LITTLE and his colleagues in Palo Alto altered the argon laser and slit-lamp so that the laser beam was directed into the slit lamp by two aluminum tubes.

1970   BYRON SMITH improved the Kuhnt-Szymanowski technique by preserving the lid margin and combining a full-thickness eyelid resection laterally with a subciliary blepharoplasty type of incision.

1970   ALSTON CALLAHAN, JOHN CLARK MUSTARDÉ and LESTER T. JONES published *Ophthalmic plastic surgery up-to-date*.

1970   J. DONALD M. GASS of Miami published his *Steroscopic atlas of macular disease*, which includes his pioneering contributions to the delineation of diseases of the retina.

1970   MARVIN H. QUICKERT (1929–1974) of San Francisco described nasolacrimal silicone intubation in the treatment of nasolacrimal duct obstruction using a bicanalicular-nasal stenting technique. In the same year, Quickert in conjunction with LESTER T. JONES and JOHN WOBIG described the cure of ptosis by aponeurotic repair.

1971   A. G. KNUDSON of Philadelphia introduced his two-hit theory on heritable and nonheritable retinoblastoma. He hypothesized that both heritable and nonheritable retinoblastoma were caused by two complementary chromosomal mutations.

1971   MICHAEL J. HOGAN and JORGE A. ALVARADO (b. 1938) published *Histology of the human eye*. The introduced their use of electron microscopy to detail histology and was accompanied by the outstanding interperative of JOAN ESPERSON WEDDELL.

1971   ROBERT MACHEMER in Miami developed a vitreous infusion suction cutter, which proved to be a major breakthrough in the area of closed vitrectomy surgery.

1971   The distribution of commercial argon laser systems was begun, and these machines soon replaced xenon photocoagulators for treating retinal lesions.

1971   GUILLERMO B. DE VENECIA (b. 1932) and coworkers at the University of Wisconsin-Madison demonstrated cytomegalic virus infection of the retina in immuno-supressed organ transplant patients.

1971   LORENZ E. ZIMMERMAN at the Armed Forces Institute of Pathology described phakomatous choristoma of the eyelid, a tumor of lenticular anlage.

1972   LESTER T. JONES and MERRILL J. REEH of Portland, Oregon published their study of lower eyelid instability and attributed the cause to weakening of the lower eyelid retractors.

1972   NORMAN S. JAFFE (b. 1924) of Miami published *Cataract surgery and its complications*.

1972   ALEX E. KRILL (1928–1972) of the University of Chicago published *Hereditary retinal and choroidal diseases*. His work provided a meaningful categorization of chorioretinal disease based on clinical tests and functional disorders.

1972   C. O'MALLEY and R. M. HEINTZ introduced their 'divided-system instrumentation' for vitrectomy via pars plana. This bimanual method offered numerous advantages, allowing greater precision for retinal surgeons.

1972   J. M. PAREL, ROBERT MACHEMER, and coworkers in Miami developed their fiberoptic intraocular illumination system for vitreal and retinal surgery.

1972   FRANCIS A. L'ESPERANCE published his clinical studies on krypton laser photocoagulation.

1972   CORNELIUS D. BINKHORST in the Netherlands devised a new intraocular lens procedure, consisting of an extracapsular cataract extraction with implantation of his iridocapsular lens into the posterior chamber. Fixation to the capsular remnant immobilized the lens and spared the corneal endothelium.

1972   MICHAEL SHEA (b. 1928) in Toronto reported the treatment of proliferative diabetic retinopathy involving transvitreal diathermy of retinal vessels.

1972   MILTON BONIUK (b. 1932) and LORENZ E. ZIMMERMAN at the Armed Forces Institute of Pathology reported their series of sebaceous carcinoma of the eye and orbit, familiarizing American ophthalmologists and pathologists with this entity.

1973   GHOLAN A. PEYMAN (b. 1937) and associates in Chicago described the use of intravitreous antibiotics for the management of bacterial endophthalmitis following cataract surgery.

1973   ENDRE A. BALASZ of Harvard, after studying the molecular structure and biological activity of polysaccharides of the intracellular matrix, patented ultrapure hyaluronic acid and its use as a substitute for vitreous during retinal detachment surgery.

1973   MIKHAIL MIKHAILOVITCH KRASNOV JR. in Moscow reported a reduction in intraocular pressure after puncturing the trabecular meshwork with the Q-switched ruby laser.

1973   JOHN WARREN HENDERSON at the Mayo Clinic published *Orbital tumors*, giving a clear and comprehensive account of the diagnosis and management of orbital tumors.

1973   D. JACKSON COLEMAN (b. 1934) at Columbia-Harkness invented a diamond knife with an edge thickness of 30 nm for use in severing vitreous strands.

1973   EDWARD W. D. NORTON reintroduced Rosengren's method of intraocular gas tamponade. Norton combined sulfur hexafluoride with air; the sulfur hexafluoride offered a slower absorption rate and potential for postoperative expansion with higher concentrations.

1973   The Douvas cataractroto-extractor, although it was designed to remove juvenile cataracts, gained popularity for closed vitrectomy due to its efficient cutting mechanisms and rugged construction.

1973   DANIEL M. ALBERT (b. 1936) at Yale University, MARK O. M. TAO at the Armed Forces Institute of Pathology, and coworkers described organ cultures of human retinal pigment epithelium (RPE) and choroids, providing a model for the study of cytological behavior of the RPE in vitro.

1974   HERMANN BURIAN of Iowa City and GUNTHER K. VON NOORDEN at the Wilmer Institue coauthored *Binocular vision and ocular motility*, explaining the mechanisms operating in ocular motility.

1974 ROBERT MACHEMER of Miami and associates invented an automated vitreous scissors and hooked needle for peeling and cutting epiretinal membranes.

1974 IAN J. CONSTABLE (b. 1943) of Australia presented his experimental results on ocular irradiation with accelerated protons.

1974 J. M. PAREL, ROBERT MACHEMER, and their colleagues introduced an operating microscope that included 'motorized, foot-controlled functions for focusing, zoom magnification, and two dimensional (X-Y) movement of the microscope head in a horizontal plane.'

1975 CHARLES KELMAN published his text *Phacoemulsification and aspiration: the Kelman technique of cataract removal.* The soon became the standard cataract procedure.

1975 The first bipolar diathermy device was described by GEORGE W. TATE (b. 1941) and associates at the University of Texas–Southwestern. The current was confined to an elliptical field between the two electrodes.

1976 JOHN PEARCE designed one of the first effective posterior chamber intraocular lenses.

1976 THOMAS D. DUANE, chairman of ophthalmology at Jefferson Medical College and ophthalmologist-in-chief at Philadelphia's Wills Eye Hospital, edited *Clinical ophthalmology.*

1976 LESTER T. JONES and JOHN L. WOBIG of Portland, Oregon, coauthored *Surgery of the eyelids and lacrimal system,* which continued to emphasize anatomical principles in modern ophthalmic plastic surgery.

1976 LARS M. VISTNES gave the first report of the 'anophthalmic socket syndrome,' which included enophthalmos of the prosthesis, a deep upper sulcus, ptosis, and lower eyelid laxity.

1976 STEVEN T. CHARLES (b. 1942) and colleagues in Memphis, Tennessee, devised a bimanual bipolar diathermy with two instruments already present in the eye serving as electrodes.

1976 ROBERT MACHEMER of Miami gave the first report of treating a macular hole with transvitreal cryotherapy.

1976 R. W. FLOWERS and B. F. HOCHHEIMER published 'Indocyanine green dye fluorescence and infrared absorption choroidal angiography performed simultaneously with fluoroscein angiography.'

1976 The National Eye Institute issued its preliminary report on the Diabetic Retinopathy Study (DRS) indicating that the benefits of photocoagulation outweigh the risks. MATTHEW D. DAVIS (b. 1926), Chair of ophthalmology at the University of Wisconsin–Madison played a major role in designing and carrying out this landmark study.

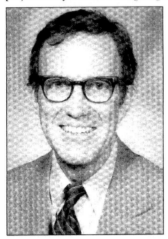

Matthew D. Davis
(b. 1926)

1976   DAVID H. ABRAMSON (b. 1944) of New York and coworkers reported that over 10% of patients who have survived treatment for bilateral retinoblastoma have developed a second monocular tumor.

1977   FREDERICK A. JAKOBIEC (b. 1942), MARK O. M. TSO, LORENZ E. ZIMMERMAN and coworkers at the Armed Forces Institute of Pathology described retinoblastoma and intracranial malignancy (trilateral retinoblastoma).

1977   THOM ZIMMERMAN and HERBERT E. KAUFMAN in New Orleans reported on the effectiveness of Timololl, a beta-adrenergic blocking agent, in the treatment of glaucoma.

1977   STEPHEN P. SHEARING introduced a compressible haptic posterior chamber intraocular lenses. Insertion was relatively easy and fixation immediately achieved.

1977   PAUL LOUIS TESSIER edited *Chirurgie plastique orbito-palpébrale*, a superb interdisciplinary monograph sponsored by the Society of Ophthalmology.

1977   JOSÉ IGNACIO BARRAQUER in Bogota, Columbia, instructed the first class on keratomileusis and keratophakia.

1977   DAVID MILLER (b. 1931) in Boston reported the use of Na-hyaluronate during intraocular lens implantation in rabbits.

1977   D. JACKSON COLEMAN at Columbia-Harkness published *Ultrasonography of the eye and orbit*, which included the presentation of much of his pioneering work in this field.

1978	DANIEL M. EICHENBAUM (b. 1942) and colleagues in Miami introduced the use of pars plana vitrectomy for the management of bacterial endophthalmitis following cataract surgery.
1978	LEO D. BORES (b. 1937) at the Kresge Institute was one of the first to perform refractive keratotomy in the United States. This followed a trip to Moscow where SVYATOSLAV FYODOROV taught him his technique.
1978	EVANGELOS S. GRAGONDAS (b. 1941) of Boston and associates published their promising primary results regarding proton irradiation of choroidal melanomas.
1979	ENDRE A. BALAZS and L. G. PAPE of Boston presented their concept of viscosurgery to the American Academy of Ophthalmology and Otolaryngology.
1979	J. WISE and S. WITTER popularized the use of argon laser as therapy for open-angle glaucoma. The lowering of intraocular tension lasts from months to years.
1979	MERRILL GRAYSON (b. 1919) of Indianapolis published *Diseases of the cornea*, a clear, beautifully illustrated introductory text to corneal disease.
1979	SVYATOSLAV N. FYODOROV in Moscow published his article that advocated treating myopia with anterior keratotomy. He proposed the use of biomechanical formulas to increase the reliability of the surgery and is credited with establishing the foundation of modern radial and astigmatic keratotomy.
1979	BENJAMIN MILDER and MELVIN L. RUBIN published their text *The fine art of prescribing glass without making a spectacle of yourself*. This introduces a light-hearted note to the too-often humorless task of learning to refract.
1979	Krypton lasers for photocoagulation became commercially available and gained popularity for subretinal neovascularization treatment close to the macula and for media opacities caused by vitreous hemorrhage or cataract.
1979	KARL C. OSSOINING (b. 1934) in Iowa City published a description of his ultrasonography unit and its use in ophthalmic diagnosis.
1979	GHOLAM A. PEYMAN of Chicago reported on his full-thickness eye wall resection of choroidal neoplasms.
1979	ALICE R. MCPHERSON of Houston reported on effectiveness of scleral buckling in infants with retinal detachment associated with retrolental fibroplasia.

1980   FRANK M. POLLACK and associates in Gainesville, Florida, reported histologic and clinical evidence regarding the protective effect of Na-hyaluronate on the corneal endothelium in intraocular surgery.

1980   Computerized (automated) perimetry became commercially available to ophthalmologists.

1980   DANIELE S. ARON-ROSA (b. 1934) of Paris initiated the use of a neodymium:YAG laser for management of secondary membranes following extracapsular cataract surgery.

1980   ALAN B. SCOTT of San Francisco introduced the injection of Botulinum A toxin into extraocular muscles as an alternative to strabismus surgery.

1980   F. FRAUNFELDER (b. 1934) of Portland, Oregon, and F. HAMPTON ROY (b. 1937) of Little Rock, Arkansas, edited *Current ocular therapy*, which briefly covers the diagnosis and treatment of almost every disease an ophthalmologist could encounter.

1980   The Prospective Evaluation of Radial Keratotomy (PERK) study was established and funded by the National Eye Institute. Radial keratotomy was critically analyzed using information gathered from university-based and private ophthalmologists and produced a wealth of information about its safety and effectiveness.

1980   HERBERT E. KAUFMAN and THEODORE P. WERBLIN (b. 1944) of New Orleans introduced aphakic epikeratoplasty designed to produce 'living contact lenses' for patients who could not wear contact lenses. The procedure involved suturing prelathed donor corneal tissue onto a deepithelialized cornea.

1980   MIGUEL F. REFOJO and his colleagues in Boston reported on a hydrophilic scleral buckling material composed of polymethyl acrylate and co-hydroxyethyl acrylate. This new material had several advantages over the standard silicone sponge and is now commonly used by retinal surgeons.

1980   JOSÉ IGNACIO BARRAQUER of Bogota described his technique for conjunctival autograft transplantation for advanced and recurrent pterygia. This procedure was modified and popularized by KENNETH R. KENYON (b. 1943) of Boston.

1981   The *Journal of Clinical Neuro-ophthalmology* was begin and edited by J. LAWTON SMITH. It later was renamed the *Journal of Neuro-ophthalmology* (1995) and became the official publication of the North American Neuro-Ophthalmology Society.

1981   JAY A. FLEISCHMANN and associates described their clinical results with a portable argon laser endophotocoagulator. PEYMAN and co-workers described their experience in the same year.

1982   BRUCE M. SHIELDS (b. 1941) of Duke University published *A study guide for glaucoma* for his students, which became popular and was expanded into the *Textbook of glaucoma* in 1987.

1982   MANUS C. KRAFF (b. 1931) of Chicago and his colleagues presented their secondary intraocular lens implantation, which they stated was useful for aphakic patients who are unable to use aphakic spectacles or contact lenses.

1982   IRVING HENRY LEOPOLD (1915–1993) of Newport Beach, California, reported on the effectiveness of topical levobunolod, a nonselective beta-blocker, in the treatment of increased intraocular pressure.

1982   The results of the National Eye Institute's Macular Photocoagulation Study (MPS) were reported. Argon laser treatment as applied in the study reduced visual acuity loss in age-related macular degeneration. The principle investigator was STUART L. FINE (b. 1942) of Baltimore.

1982   BRENDA L. GALLIE (b. 1944) in Toronto and associates described 'retinoma,' a benign variant of retinoblastoma. The following year, CURTIS E. MARGO and coworkers at the Armed Forces Institute of Pathology independently described this tumor and term it 'retinocytoma.'

1983   HENRY I. BAYLIS (b. 1935) and R. TOBY SUTCLIFFE reported on their retroseptal approach to transconjunctival blepharoplasty. The current popularity of the transconjunctival approach is attributed to their technique.

1983   MARSHALL M. PARKS and his colleagues from the Children's Hospital in Washington, D.C., introduced the usage of posterior lens capsulectomy and automated anterior vitrectomy for surgery in children with cataracts. This surgery resulted in less frequent occurrence of amblyopia due to secondary membranes.

1983   *Ophthalmic Plastic and Reconstructive Surgery* was founded and published quarterly with HENRY I. BAYLIS of Los Angeles as editor. BERNICE Z. BROWN (b. 1931) of Los Angeles and RICHARD K. DORTZBACH (b. 1936) of Madison, Wisconsin, were subsequent editors.

1983   The excimer laser was introduced to clinical ophthalmology and used to reshape the cornea by photorefraction. This technology is currently used in the PRK and LASIK procedures.

1983   JOHN LEIGH and DAVID S. ZEE co-authored *The neurology of the eye*. The book focuses on the clinical aspects of disorders of eye movements.

1983   CHARLES L. SCHEPENS of Boston published *Retinal detachment and allied diseases*, which gives a broad view of retinal detachment surgery and includes the many advances made by the Schepens group.

1983   JERRY SHIELDS (b. 1937) of Wills Eye Hospital published *Diagnosis and management of orbital tumors* based on his vast clinical experience in ocular oncology.

1983   R. SLOAN WILSON of Little Rock, Arkansas, reported his clinical and experimental research on the use of synthetic absorbable scleral buckling materials, including polyglactin 910, polyglycolic acid, and polydioxanone.

1983   A. RAY IRVINE JR. (b. 1938) and H. R. McDONALD of San Francisco described light-induced maculopathy resulting from the operating microscope in extracapsular lens extraction and intraocular lens implantation.

1983   Additional results of the Macular Photocoagulation Study indicate the usefulness of argon laser treatment in presumed ocular histoplasmosis and neovascular membranes.

1984   MICHAEL G. GRESSEL, RICHARD K. PARRISH II, and ROBERT FOLBERG reported on the use of 5-fluorouracil in glaucoma filtering surgery in an animal model.

1984   SAMUEL PACKER (b. 1941) at North Shore University published his favorable clinical results in iodine-125 irradiation of choroidal melanoma.

1984   D. J. SPALTON, R. A. HITCHINGS, and P. A. HUNTER published *Atlas of clinical ophthalmology*.

1985   WILLIAM SPENCER (b. 1925) of San Francisco edited a totally rewritten, *Ophthalmic pathology*.

1986   THADEUS DRYJA, STEVEN FRIEND, and associates in Boston cloned the

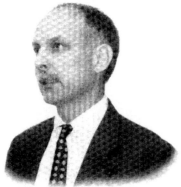

Thadeus Dryja

retinoblastoma gene, a major advance in cancer genetics.

1987   HARRY W. FLYNN JR. (b. 1945) and his colleagues in Miami presented their results using pars plana lensectomy and vitrectomy in the treatment of complicated cataract patients with juvenile rheumatoid arthritis.

1987   The first report of the National Eye Institute's Early Treatment Diabetic Retinopathy Study (ETDRS) is published. Photocoagulation reduced the risk of moderate vision, especially in eyes with macular edema. Aspirin did not affect the pregression of retinopathy.

1989   HUMPHRIES and his associates in Ireland, following the candidate gene method, mapped the mutated gene in a family with autosomal-dominant retinitis pigmentosa.

1989   HENRY D. JAMPEL (b. 1956) and coworkers reported on initial trials of aproclonidine in the treatment of glaucoma. This drug showed effective pressure lowering and reasonable safety but high pharmacologic tolerance.

1989   STEPHEN J. RYAN (b. 1940) in Los Angeles edited *Retina*, one of the outstanding texts for the subspecialty of vitreo-retinal ophthalmology.

1989   CARL B. CAMRAS and associates reported on maintained reduction of intraocular pressure by prostaglandin F_2-1-isopropyl ester in glaucoma patients, an important milestone in the development of latanoprost treatment.

1990   THADEUS DRYJA and associates in Boston were the first to clone and sequence a mutated gene responsible for retinitis pigmentosa.

1990   HOWARD V. GIMBEL (b. 1934) of Calgary and T. NEUHANN of Munich reported on the continuous circular capsulorhexis technique for intraocular lens implantation.

1990   STEVEN M. PODOS (b. 1937) of New York and coworkers reported the encouraging results of clinical trials studying the effectiveness of the topical carbonic anhydrase inhibitor dorzolamide to lower intraocular pressure in humans.

1993   IRENE E. LOEWENFELD of New York published *The pupil: anatomy, physiology and clinical applications* based upon the research of herself and her husband, OTTO LÖWENSTEIN (1890–1965).

1994   The Eye Bank Association of America reported that the number of corneal transplants done in the United States had risen to 44,000.

1994   HAROLD RIDLEY was presented the Gonin Medal for his contributions to the field of ophthalmology, particularly the invention of the intraocular lens.

1994   DANIEL M. ALBERT of Madison, Wisconsin, and FREDERICK A. JACOBIEC (b. 1942), both ophthalmic pathologists, published their comprehensive *Principles and practice of ophthalmology*.

1995   ARTHUR POLANS (b. 1953) and associates in Portland, Oregon demonstrated that recoverin, a photoreceptor-specific calcium binding protein is expressed by tumors and is a presumed etiologic factor in cancer associated retinopathy (CAR).

1996   The fourth edition of *Ophthalmic pathology* was published under the editorship of WILLIAM SPENCER of San Francisco.

1997   JAY H. KRACHMER (b. 1941) of Minneapolis, MARK MANNIS (b. 1946) of Sacramento, and EDWARD J. HOLLAND (b. 1946) published *Cornea*. It is the most comprehensive current work on fundamentals, diagnosis, and management of corneal disease

1997   CLAES H. DOHLMAN of Boston published his experience with keratoprostheses indicating improved results from previous reports.

2000   The Rabb-Venable Ophthalmology Award for Outstanding Research was founded as a tribute to MAURICE F. RABB and H. PHILLIP VENABLE. Rabb and Venable were the first African-Americans to serve as namesakes for an academic research award.

2002   The results of the medium-sized tumor arm of the Collaborative Ocular Melanoma Study were published. Enucleation and I^{125} bracytherapy had equivalent survival statistics.

Printed and bound by CPI Group (UK) Ltd, Croydon, CR0 4YY

23/10/2024

01778242-0008